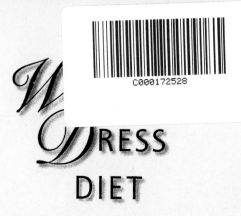

WEDDING DRESS DIET

Robyn Flipse is a registered dietitian who is frequently quoted in such publications as *Cosmopolitan* and *Good Housekeeping* and is a regular guest on US health and nutrition television programmes. She lives in New Jersey.

Jacqueline Shannon is the author of thirteen books as well as having written articles for numerous US magazines including *Cosmopolitan*, for which she was a regular columnist. She lives in San Diego.

Visit the *Wedding Dress Diet* website:
www. *wedding dress diet.com*.

THE WEDDING DRESS DIET

Robyn Flipse, R.D.
and Jacqueline Shannon

ARROW

Published by Arrow Books in 2000

1 3 5 7 9 10 8 6 4 2

Copyright © Robyn Flipse and Jacqueline Shannon 2000

Robyn Flipse and Jacqueline Shannon have asserted their
right under the Copyright, Designs and Patents Act, 1988 to
be identified as the authors of this work

First published in the United Kingdom in 2000 by Arrow

Arrow Books
The Random House Group Limited
20 Vauxhall Bridge Road, London, SW1V 2SA

The Random House Group Limited supports The Forest Stewardship
Council (FSC®), the leading international forest certification organisation.
Our books carrying the FSC label are printed on FSC® certified paper.
FSC is the only forest certification scheme endorsed by the leading
environmental organisations, including Greenpeace. Our
paper procurement policy can be found at
www.randomhouse.co.uk/environment

Random House Group Limited Reg. No. 954009
www.randomhouse.co.uk

A CIP catalogue record for this book
is available from the British Library

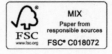

MIX
Paper from
responsible sources
FSC® C018072

ISBN13: 9780099542629

Design/make up by Roger Walker

Printed and bound in Great Britain by Clays Ltd, St Ives PLC

Addresses for companies within The Random House Group Limited can be found
www.randomhouse.co.uk/offices.htm

To my son, Peter Samuel Flipse Dorian
Robyn Flipse

To my daughter, Madeline Maria Trobaugh
Jacqueline Shannon

Contents

★ Calculating your exercise heart rate
★ Counting calories isn't enough: how to
shape, tone and define your features
★ The truth about cellulite
★ Why it's great to have an exercise buddy
★ Choosing a gym, personal trainer and more
★ Posture pointers: how to 'lose' five pounds
in one minute
★ Exercise myths and realities
★ Calorie burners and toners you can do while
you're doing other things

6 EATING BETWEEN FITTINGS ★ 143
★ Danger: skipping meals
★ Eating on the run or on the road: best choices
at the fast-food restaurant, supermarket,
convenience store and more

7 SHOWERED WITH CALORIES ★ 157
★ Keeping your head – and your diet – at all
of the parties thrown in your honour including
the hen night!
★ Special tips for safely navigating a buffet and
surviving 'samplings' at the caterer's

8 SETTING UP A SLIM KITCHEN ★ 175
★ Slim-conscious cookware and gadgets
★ Stocking the pantry
★ Recommended cookbooks, magazines,
websites and more

Wedding Dress Woes

Two weeks before her June wedding, twenty-eight-year-old Sarah Williams* went for the final fitting of her wedding dress. As she stood on a raised platform for the seamstress, Sarah was horrified to see that her stomach bulged out quite noticeably in the clinging, floor-length tube of a slip dress she had chosen.

*name changed at her insistence

*S*arah called this to the attention of her mother and the seamstress. The seamstress clucked her tongue sympathetically. 'You could always wear control briefs,' she said, heading off to find what our mothers used to call a girdle so that Sarah could see just how much her pot-belly could be masked. The 'tummy terminator' nearly took Sarah's breath away with its industrial-strength Lycra. Worse, the pot-belly was still apparent.

Sarah's mother sighed heavily. 'That's what you get for ordering a dress six months in advance.'

'Like I had a choice,' Sarah snapped, glaring at her mother. But when she got home and stepped on the scales, she realised her mother had a point. She'd put on several lbs.* She couldn't lay the blame entirely on the glasses of champagne she'd downed at various pre-marriage celebrations with her friends, nor the 'Mexican and Margherita' extravanganza of her hen night the week before. Forced to run around seeing to all the details of her huge, elaborate wedding during her lunch hours, for the past few months Sarah had been opting for fast-food lunches . . .

---

*All references to body weight are given in Imperial measures. For metric equivalents please see conversion chart on page 21

Well, Sarah vowed, this was war. She had two weeks to battle her bulge. She did some research on the Internet, scanning the archives of women's magazines for diets that promised to help a reader lose 10 lbs in two weeks or less. She settled on an extreme version of what's commonly known as the Dr Atkins diet. She ate vast quantities of protein and some fat, but zero carbohydrates.

For two weeks, Sarah ate nothing but meat and cheese.

No carbohydrates. No vegetables or fruit. Water weight poured off of her. She was constantly in the bathroom. Within 11 days, she'd lost 11 lbs. Two days before the wedding, however, she woke up with a painful, swollen tongue. It hurt to talk. It hurt to swallow. She visited her doctor. 'It's either a virus that will go away in a few days, or your diet has been very poor,' the doctor told her.

When her wedding day arrived, Sarah's tongue still hurt. She could barely find the energy to walk down the aisle. She was so exhausted that she and her new husband had to leave their expensive, carefully planned reception much earlier than they'd expected. On her Hawaiian honeymoon, Sarah indulged herself in breads, rice, pasta, potatoes – all the carbohydrates she'd been craving. She felt bloated on the beach in Maui and refused to let her new husband take pictures of her in her bikini.

***Back in England Sarah discovered she'd
regained every bit of the weight she had
struggled to lose . . . and more!***

Sarah grins sheepishly when she relates this tale, then
tells us a friend of hers – let's call her Lisa – can top it. Lisa
was so desperate to lose 10 lbs in the week before her
own wedding that she went to a seven-day, boot-camp-
like 'fasting' camp in which only water was served. By the
fourth day, Lisa was so starving that she stole a packet of
honey from the staff dining room and brushed her teeth
with it, spitting it out so that the medical supervisors
wouldn't catch on to her cheating.

Professionally, we, the authors, have heard dozens
of similar horror stories – Robyn, as a registered dietitian who has maintained a thriving nutrition coun-
selling practice for 15 years, and Jacqueline, a long-
time freelance health writer who not too long ago
wrote both the health and diet columns for American
Cosmopolitan.

The typical bride-to-be's desperate vow – 'I must
look perfect on my wedding day' – is a mantra we've
often heard in our personal lives as well. Within the last
year Robyn participated in two weddings, once as
mother of the groom, once as sister of the bride. Jacqueline was twice a bridesmaid. Earlier in our lives, each of
us was a bride. We know that the size label in a woman's
wedding dress is a number that will live with her forever.
(And she's got the photos and videotapes to prove it!)
Years later, she may not remember the names of all of her

bridesmaids, but she *will* remember whether she was a size 10 or a size 20 as she took her vows.

And who can blame women for obsessing about wanting to look the best they'll ever look at this pinnacle event? After all,

a woman's wedding day is the one day in her life she's guaranteed to be the star of the show,

the centre of attention, the person in the spotlight. All eyes will be on her.

Even celebrities who are accustomed to living their lives under the constant scrutiny of the public eye feel a special paranoia about their wedding day. In the weeks before her wedding to Prince Edward, Sophie Rhys-Jones, for example, underwent a bizarre treatment called a 'Frigi-Thalgo' body wrap in order to help her lose 20 lbs. If you can believe the tabloid press, Sophie was 'smeared with a foul-smelling seaweed concoction and then wrapped mummy-style in cold, wet bandages'. It's 'a bit like sitting in your wet clothes after you come in from the rain'. Except that you stink, too.

Sarah Ferguson recently recalled the drastic steak-and-oranges diet she tried the month before her wedding. She rounded out those deadly boring diet meals with 'injections and pills – and we're not talking vitamins either,' she said. 'Your hair falls out and your skin's a mess, but you lose weight! I lost 26 lbs in 4 weeks.'

Not long after, the 5ft 8in duchess ballooned to 15 stone.

Do we believe that women are far too hard on them-selves when it comes to body image? Absolutely! Do we also accept the reality that almost all brides-to-be go on a diet? That too! One of us – Robyn – can document the fact that prospective brides are the third-largest group of people (after athletes and pregnant women) concerned about their weight.

Our mission is this: with our safe and sane diet and exercise plan, we will help you, the soon-to-be-married woman, accomplish your weight-loss and shape-up goals without sacrificing your skin or your hair or your energy or your sanity for, say, your thunder thighs. In addition, our advice will keep your immune system healthy and strong so you can survive all of the stress of getting to the church on time.

The corollary to this is you will have the foundation for a varied and healthy eating style for life. You have probably heard the statistic that '95 per cent of all diets fail'. This is misleading; it implies you can't lose weight on a diet. The truth is that most people *do* lose weight when they go on a diet. But 95 per cent of them put the weight back on within a year. That's mostly thanks to the rigidity and monotony of the majority of diets.

Sure, you can eat nothing but steak and oranges for a couple of weeks – but think about staying on that diet for the next year!

You couldn't! You would go absolutely mad! You would crave the forbidden so much that one day, like a crazed animal, you would wrestle that package of chocolate digestives from your new husband's hands and – spitting and snarling – devour the entire packet without even bothering to sit down. Sooner rather than later, you would balloon just like Fergie and you'd become a card-carrying member of the '95 Per cent Club'.

That won't happen here. There is nothing monotonous about *The Wedding Dress Diet*.

Our philosophy is that you can eat anything you want . . . in moderation.

Moderation meaning that if you split a dish of chocolate mousse with your best friend at lunch, then don't have dessert after dinner. Because in our book, calories are king. It's not the proverbial end-all and be-all – Robyn is, after all, a dietitian with some very hardcore beliefs about good nutrition (as you'll learn in Chapter Four). But we live in the real world, too. We know the odds of finding a bag of baby carrots in your office vending machine as opposed to a Mars bar or bag of Doritos. So you won't get a lot of finger wagging from us. You blow it occasionally? In our book, the day is still salvageable – you'll have no excuse to say, 'Well, since I blew it at lunch I might as well go all out at dinner, too.'

The Wedding Dress Diet is not monotonous, but it is rigid . . . especially if, like Fergie, you have blessed few weeks left until your big day. We are going to coach you to be hyperstrict about calories and exercising during the weeks or months you are dieting. You have to be, because unlike most dieters, you have a hard and fast deadline for losing the weight: your wedding day. What makes our plan special, however, is that you get to decide on the relative rigidity of your personal plan. We provide a simple formula to enable you to determine exactly how many calories you must limit yourself to eating each day and how much exercising you must do based on the weeks or months till your wedding and the number of lbs you want to lose. Another silver lining of *The Wedding Dress Diet* is that we give you lots and lots of tips and guidelines so that, even after you've reached your goal weight and can loosen up on your calorie and exercise quotas, you can eat deliciously and nutritiously while maintaining your weight loss forever and without feeling deprived, or hungry, or simply bored to death.

There are lots of other features in this diet book which make it different from any others. For example:

♥ We'll help you cope with this unique predicament: While you may feel that, say, the four months you have remaining until your wedding is ample time to reach your goal weight, you may be stunned to discover that you must order your wedding gown at least four to six months in advance . . . that is, well before you achieve the body you want!

♥ With our chapter on selecting the right wedding dress, we will not leave out advice for you if, for whatever reason, you have not achieved the body you were hoping for before your wedding. With our suggestions on selecting the perfect neckline, skirt style, and so on, we will show you how to maximise your particular figure assets while minimising those you're not happy with.

♥ We are also very democratic. We recognise that most of our readers will be first-time brides, but we don't forget the second-time-around bride. In our exercise chapter, for example, we address the needs of the woman who is working on her second wedding and who may not have much time or energy for working out because she may be juggling not just a top-flight career but a couple of kids, as well. Another example: in our chapter on selecting the perfect wedding dress, we don't merely help brides mask common but changeable problems, such as a protruding tummy, but also those who have irreversible 'flaws', such as being very short in stature.

♥ Finally, we won't abandon you at the altar! Our book takes you well beyond your wedding day. We provide not just simple, delicious ways to maintain your new figure for years to come but also tips on such topics as how to indulge but not overdo it on your honeymoon and how to get your husband and your in-laws to adapt – or at least tolerate and support – your new healthy lifestyle.

Congratulations on your engagement.
And now, let's go, girl!

CHAPTER ONE
Taking Stock

Ask any woman if she is happy with her body and she will undoubtedly say 'No', and then proceed to list the usual figure flaws. But for a bride-to-be, figure flaws seem to become a matter of life and death. No one wants to walk down the aisle, all eyes upon her, with 'thunder thighs', 'a pot belly', and/or 'flabby arms'. Fortunately, no one has to.

*B*y now you've probably figured out that the perfect wedding takes lots of time and heaps of planning. If so, you're making daily 'to-do' lists and checking them twice. Fitting into the perfect gown takes the same strategy.

A series of fad diets interspersed with bouts of manic exercise will not help you get into shape for your big day

or stay in shape for a minute after. You need a more personal approach to lose your unwanted lbs and firm those reluctant muscles.

If you are ready to commit to an eating and exercise overhaul, you will reap endless benefits. Try to think of *The Wedding Dress Diet* as a new part-time job. Yes, it's more work for you at a time when you're already madly busy, but the payoff is also like a second income. You will look and feel great, and can continue to collect the dividends as long as you do the work.

As with any new job, there's some paperwork to complete. In this case, it is working out what your body measurements are now. Then you can follow the chapter-by-chapter instructions that will help you change your size and shape into something you'll be proud to have captured in all those wedding photos.

Taking inventory of your vital statistics

In the privacy of your bedroom or bathroom, you must face the brutal truth.

Strip down to your birthday suit and take these all-important measurements to use as a baseline of where you are now and where you hope to get to in the months ahead. You will need:

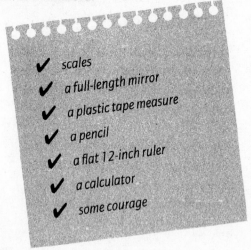

- ✔ scales
- ✔ a full-length mirror
- ✔ a plastic tape measure
- ✔ a pencil
- ✔ a flat 12-inch ruler
- ✔ a calculator
- ✔ some courage

Forget all those excuses for why the scales aren't right. It doesn't matter if they give a different reading from the scales in the gym or your doctor's office. What matters is that each week you will return to your scales and record the change of weight they report. Do not get on the scales more than once a week. Body weight fluctuates from morning to night due to changes in hydration and elimination. Your weight will also fluctuate at different times throughout your menstrual cycle. This is normal. What you need to focus on are the changes in weight over time that are permanent, not transient.

Body weight is not the most important, or revealing, aspect of your appearance anyway. No one else actually gets to see the number on your scales. What people notice about you is the way you carry and present yourself. It's the total package. Posture and proportions are big parts of that image, along with height and weight. You can do very little about how tall you are, but you can look taller and thinner with better posture and certain fashion choices. You can definitely reshape proportions through weight loss (or gain) and exercise. See Chapters Three, Five and Six for more advice on these changes.

The weigh-in

Place your scales on a flat surface–preferably not on carpet or tiles. If you're using floor-model scales with a numerical readout, set the dial so that the arrow points directly at zero. For digital scales, be sure the battery is new and the LED panel is blank (or zero) when first turned on. If you're using balance-beam scales, slide the top and bottom weights to zero to ensure that the bar is balanced with nothing on the scales. Now step on to the scales and record exactly what you weigh in lbs. (Use the chart on pages 24–25 to record this – and other measurements – today and again before the wedding.)

Your true height

Find a section of wall that rises from an uncarpeted floor and has no obstructions at the base, such as a molding or heating panel. Grab your pencil and ruler. Stand barefooted with your back against the wall and your legs together. Be sure the backs of your heels, buttocks, shoulders and head are touching the wall.

Place the ruler on your head so one end touches the wall and the other extends over your forehead. Position the ruler so it is balanced, then gently press down on the centre of the ruler on top of your head. Hold the pencil in your other hand and draw a line on the wall at the point where the ruler touches it.

Step away from the wall and, using the tape measure, measure the distance between the line you drew and the floor directly below it. Convert the measurement to inches by multiplying each foot by 12, then add any remaining inches to that for your total.

Top-to-bottom circumference measurements

Take all of the following measurements while naked. We realise that one or more of these 'parts' may not show when you're wearing your wedding dress – but they will on your honeymoon!

★ **Bust** – (Grab one end of the flexible plastic tape measure and wrap it around your back before grabbing the other end in your free hand. Stand sideways and look into the mirror while pulling the tape up towards your armpits. Stop at the point on your back opposite the natural protrusion of your breasts. Gently pull the end of the tape over your nipples and take a reading of the inches around your bustline.

★ **Waist** – Drop the tape down to below your ribs and above your hips where your body indents the most. Don't inhale or deliberately flatten your stomach. Exhale and take a reading of the inches around your waistline.

★ **Hips** – Looking sideways into the mirror, lower the tape so it rides over the most protruding part of your behind. Wrap the tape around, so it encircles you without rising up in the front. Take a reading of the inches around your hips.

★ **Thigh** (Get help, if available, for this measurement.) – Stand with your feet shoulder-width apart and your weight evenly distributed over each foot. Bending slightly at the waist, wrap the tape around your right leg at the thickest, uppermost part and take a reading. Now measure the left thigh. Be sure you do not bend your knees or tighten the muscles in your leg while measuring your thighs.

★ **Calf** (Get help, if available, for this measurement.) – Stand with your weight evenly distributed on both feet and shoulder-width apart. Measure the distance between your ankle bone on the side of your foot and the crease in back of your knee. Find the mid-point between these two spots and wrap the tape around your calf for a measurement.

★   **Upper Arm** (Get help, if available, for this measurement.) – Raise one arm at a time directly in front of you, with palm facing up, until your extended arm is level with your shoulder. Measure the distance between the crease in your elbow and your shoulder bone. Find the midpoint between these two spots and wrap the tape around your arm, without flexing the muscle, for a measurement.

★   **Frame** – Extend the thumb and index finger of your dominant hand as if making a gun. Place your opposite wrist into the crotch of your extended fingers, then wrap your thumb and index finger around your wrist to the point at which they meet. Be sure you use only your thumb and index finger to encircle your wrist. If your thumb and index finger *overlap*, you have a *small frame*. If they *just meet*, you have a *medium frame*. If they *don't touch*, you have a *large frame*. Frame size is largely determined by the size and configuration of your bones, so it's not going to change if you lose weight. However, it's important to know your frame size because height-weight charts are often further categorised by frame size. In other words, if you're 5ft 8in with a large frame, your 'healthy weight' range will be higher than that of a woman who is the same height but who possesses a smaller frame.

Surreal versus ideal weight

There is no law against dreaming, but let's face it: you have only a few months until the wedding.

At best you can expect to lose
2–3 lbs a week.

More likely, you will average 1 or 2 lbs a week.

On the following pages, we've included two different methods for helping you determine a *healthy* weight for your size; and the definition of 'healthy' here is what places you at lowest risk of developing and/or succumbing to underweight conditions, such as osteoporosis and amenorrhoea (loss of menstrual periods), and those most common in the obese, diabetes and high blood pressure. First, you'll find a height-weight chart, further categorised by frame size. To convert lbs into stone, divide by 14. To convert into kilograms, divide by 2.2. These are good, general guidelines used by life insurance companies. The chief criticism against charts of this type, however, is that the data comes from people who are buying life insurance, not from a representative sample of the population. In other words, such charts don't take into account socio-economic or ethnic differences among people which can be a factor when it comes to so-called 'ideal weights'. For example, a typical African-American tends to have a heavier skeletal frame, though this in itself does not put him or her at any additional

Metropolitan Life height-weight table for women

Height Feet	Inches	Small Frame (lbs)	Medium Frame (lbs)	Large Frame (lbs)
4	9	99–108	106–118	115–124
4	10	100–110	108–120	117–131
4	11	101–112	110–123	119–134
5	0	103–115	112–126	122–137
5	1	105–118	115–129	125–140
5	2	108–121	118–132	128–144
5	3	111–124	121–135	131–148
5	4	114–127	124–138	134–152
5	5	117–130	127–141	137–156
5	6	120–133	130–144	140–160
5	7	123–136	133–147	143–164
5	8	126–139	136–150	146–167
5	9	129–142	139–153	149–170
5	10	132–145	142–156	152–173
5	11	135–148	145–159	155–176

These ranges are for women ages 25–59 based on lowest mortality rates (that is, death!).

Source: Society of Actuaries and Association of Life Insurance Medical Directors of America.

Determining Body Mass Index (BMI)

Take the following steps, or consult the chart on pages 22–23.

Step One: Multiply your weight in lbs by 705.

Step Two: Divide the answer by your height in inches.

Step Three: Again divide that number by your height.

Example: Weight: 140 lbs

Height: 65 inches

140 multiplied by 705 = 98,700

98,700 divided by 65 = 1,518

1,518 divided by 65 = 23, the BMI

Conversion table

To Convert	Multiply by
Inches to Centimetres	2.5400
Centimetres to Inches	0.3937
Feet to Metres	0.3048
Metres to Feet	3.2810
Pounds to Kilograms	0.4536
Kilograms to Pounds	2.2050

Determining BMI by height and weight measurements

Body Mass Index:	19	20	21	22	23
Height (inches)	Body weight (lbs)				
58	91	96	100	105	110
59	94	99	104	108	113
60	97	102	107	112	118
61	100	106	111	116	122
62	104	109	115	120	126
63	107	113	118	124	130
64	110	116	122	128	134
65	114	120	126	132	138
66	118	124	130	136	142
67	121	127	134	140	146
68	125	131	138	144	151
69	128	135	142	149	155
70	132	139	146	153	160
71	136	143	150	157	165
72	140	147	154	162	169
73	144	151	159	166	174

24	25	26	27	28	29	30
115	119	124	129	134	138	143
118	123	128	133	138	143	148
123	128	133	138	143	148	153
127	132	137	143	148	153	158
131	136	142	147	153	158	164
135	141	146	152	158	163	169
140	145	151	157	163	169	174
144	150	156	162	168	174	180
148	155	161	167	173	179	186
153	159	166	172	178	185	191
158	164	171	177	184	190	197
162	169	176	182	189	196	203
167	174	181	188	195	202	207
172	179	186	193	200	208	215
177	184	191	199	206	213	221
182	189	197	204	212	219	227

Record your measurements

List your current measurements in the charts on the left; save the charts on the right for recording your measurements at a date closer to your wedding, so that you can see your progress.

Date: _____

Weight: _____

Height: _____

Bust: _____

Waist: _____

Hips: _____

Thigh: Left _____ Right _____

Calf: Left _____ Right _____

Upper arm: Left _____ Right _____

Frame (tick): ☐ small ☐ medium ☐ large

BMI: _____

Notes: _____

_____

_____

_____

_____

Date: _____

Weight: _____

Height: _____

Bust: _____

Waist: _____

Hips: _____

Thigh: Left _____ Right _____

Calf: Left _____ Right _____

Upper arm: Left _____ Right _____

Frame (tick): ☐ small ☐ medium ☐ large

BMI: _____

Notes: _____

_____

_____

_____

_____

Record your sizes

Date: _____

Shoe: _____

Hat: _____

Skirt: _____

Blouse: _____

Jacket: _____

Dress: _____

Bra: _____

Ring: _____

Gloves: _____

Trousers: _____

Coat: _____

Jeans: _____

Swimsuit: _____

Knickers: _____

Tights/stockings: _____

Other: _____

_____

_____

Date: _____

Shoe: _____

Hat: _____

Skirt: _____

Blouse: _____

Jacket: _____

Dress: _____

Bra: _____

Ring: _____

Gloves: _____

Trousers: _____

Coat: _____

Jeans: _____

Swimsuit: _____

Knickers: _____

Tights/stockings: _____

Other: _____

_____

_____

risk of succumbing to obesity-related conditions than a typical Caucasian. Therefore, an African-American's weight may be heavier than, but still as healthy, as what is indicated in the chart. For this and other similar reasons, doctors often don't agree on the cut-off points for 'healthy' versus 'unhealthy' ranges.

Our other – and the newer – guideline for helping you determine a healthy weight is the Body Mass Index, or BMI. It's now preferred by most experts, but like the height-weight charts, doctors don't always agree on the healthy versus unhealthy cut-off points. For our purposes, however, keep this general guideline in mind: a desirable BMI in women is less than 25; you're overweight if your BMI is 25 to 30, and you're obese if your BMI is above 30.

Although the weight goals represented in these charts may not be the same as your desired or ideal weight, it is important to have some idea of your weight range for good health.

CHAPTER TWO

Hide and Seek . . .

Your Best and Worst Features

Life isn't a fairy tale. When the Evil Queen in *Snow White* looked into the mirror and asked, 'Who's the fairest of them all?' she was told just what she wanted to hear. And, as we all know, that bit of misinformation didn't help her self-improvement programme one bit!

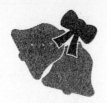

Reflections

If you live in the real world, you need to take a long, hard look into a full-length mirror and face the bare facts reflected back at you. While many aspects of your figure and your overall appearance can be changed through diet and exercise, some things cannot, no matter how hard you try. Height is one example, the shape and bone structure of your face is another.

There is hope for your unalterable features, though, and we don't mean surgery. Styling changes – in dress, in hairstyle, in make-up – have been used by actors for centuries to create illusions. Just take a close look at entertainer Ru Paul, the grand master (madam?) of deception! If men can make up to look like glamorous women, women can do it even better.

Complete the Mirror, Mirror charts on pages 32–33 to establish realistic goals for yourself. You will feel much more satisfied if you focus on things you can change, and see some results for your efforts, as opposed to going after the impossible and constantly feeling frustrated (which can, among other things, lead to overeating).

To get started on your diet and exercise changes, you must also take a realistic look at the calendar and your daily appointment book. How many weeks do you have

'Mirror, Mirror On The Wall'

Features you can change with diet and exercise

	Satisfied	Unsatisfied	Fantasy Goal	Realistic Goal
Weight	☐	☐	_____	_____
Bust*	☐	☐	_____	_____
Waist	☐	☐	_____	_____
Hips*	☐	☐	_____	_____
Stomach	☐	☐	_____	_____
Thighs	☐	☐	_____	_____
Calves	☐	☐	_____	_____
Upper arms	☐	☐	_____	_____
Neck	☐	☐	_____	_____
Posture	☐	☐	_____	_____

*Some reduction and reshaping of the bust and trimming of the hips is possible, but don't expect major renovations in these areas. Use the style pointers in Chapter 3 to further minimise or accentuate these features.

until the wedding? And how many hours per week can you dedicate to serious exercise? You will need these numbers to complete *The Wedding Dress Diet* 'Worksheet' in Chapter Four.

Features you can improve with styling

	Satisfied	Unsatisfied	Fantasy Goal	Realistic Goal
Hair colour	☐	☐	___	___
Hair length	☐	☐	___	___
Eyebrows	☐	☐	___	___
Complexion	☐	☐	___	___
Face shape	☐	☐	___	___
Facial features	☐	☐	___	___
Torso length	☐	☐	___	___
Bust*	☐	☐	___	___
Shoulder width	☐	☐	___	___
Hips*	☐	☐	___	___
Leg length	☐	☐	___	___

Features you can't do anything about

Height	HOAX shape (see Chapter 3)
Frame	Shoe size

Styling changes may not take months to accomplish, but you should allow plenty of time to phase them into your life and look. The groom shouldn't do a double-take when you reach his side because your appearance has changed so dramatically he doesn't recognise you. Remember:

stunning is good, shocking is not.

Talk to a good hairstylist about colour, cut and style possibilities, keeping in mind your headdress. Start growing out your layered look or begin trimming those long tresses so you have time to settle into your new 'do'. Many hairstylists say that hair looks best a week after you've had it cut, so keep that in mind when you make your pre-wedding appointment.

This is a good time to start thinking about your eyebrows, too. Does the colour of your brows match your hair? Will you be tweezing them into thin arcs or going for a more natural look?

It's a good idea to ask your hairstylist to give you a trial run a month before your wedding. Then jog around the block with your new style; it'll be no more taxing than the workout you'll put it through on the day of your wedding and reception. We know one bride who not only put her hairstylist through a trial run, but her make-up artist, too. (Her concern about the make-up artist is understandable when you know that she hired the woman who had done the make-up for the 'dead' people floating in the water in *Titanic*! By the way, the make-up of this thoroughly alive bride looked fabulous on her wedding day.)

If you'll be doing your own make-up, go to cosmetic counters in department stores for free advice on skincare and make-up application. You may even be able to get a free makeover at some counters. Again, give yourself plenty of time to get used to applying your make-up to highlight your bone structure while masking dark circles and other liabilities. See Chapter Three for tips.

You should also read Chapter Three before you even think about shopping for your wedding dress. Take this book with you into the bridal salons to ensure that you select the most flattering gown for your figure. It is tempting, the minute you get engaged, to start flicking through the pages of bridal magazines and window shopping for a dress. But this can be dangerous! You risk falling madly in love with the wrong gown (almost as bad as falling for the wrong man!). Unless you're committed to wearing an heirloom dress that has been in your family for years, *don't even look* at a wedding dress until you know exactly what you need to flatter your figure.

A vow to lose

Most people greatly underestimate how difficult it really is to lose 5 lbs. When you have even more than that to lose, it can be one of the toughest jobs you'll ever tackle. But it is doable. What it takes is unwavering focus and unyielding commitment – *not* will-power. What's the difference? Will-power is a short-lived emotion, such as being in love with capri pants while they're in fashion,

CHEWING THE FAT ONLINE

You're dying for a Mars bar. And you've just discovered that your flatmate stashed a warehouse-store-sized box of them in the vegetable bin of the refrigerator. Slam the door and head for your computer. While the Internet is littered with weight-loss junk – mostly pitches for particular products – there are places to go if all you want is support. One option is 'buddy boards' – electronic bulletin boards where dieters can find others who want to exchange e-mail encouragement. 'Having someone I can share advice, confessions and motivation with has made all the difference,' a woman whose online name is SOONSLIM told *Cosmo.*

If you're on America Online, find a cyberbuddy in the Thrive@Shape area.

If you're not on AOL, there are still plenty of online support sites. Author Pam Dixon, who has written five Internet guides and has also lost considerable weight herself, recommends the following:

★ **Usenet News Groups**
  alt.support.diet
  Says Dixon: 'The messages are very supportive. You can learn a lot from other people's experiences.'

★ **Web Pages**
  www.spessart.com/users/ggraham.weight.htm
  'Mostly messaging with a couple of chats. Gail Graham created the page because she couldn't find support

elsewhere on the Web. One of the many features on this site is the "Diet Crisis Center", where you can leave urgent messages and get immediate support.'

★ **Diettalk**
www.diettalk.com
'You'll find recipes and success stories here, but this is mainly a well-organised live chat page with lots of good information from experts like nutritionists, nurses and authors.'

★ **Overeaters Recovery Group Home Page**
www.hiwaay.net/recovery
'Many participants on this page are members of Overeaters Anonymous, but you don't have to be a member to participate, and the page has no official affiliation with OA. Most popular and famous (an Internet legend!), the Rosanne loop, a giant support group on compulsive overeating. It's been around forever.'

★ **Shape Up America's Support Center**
http://www.shapeup.org
This is one we found ourselves. 'Shape Up America' is a programme instituted by ex-Surgeon General C Everett Koop. Part of this excellent site on healthy eating and exercise is a support line, where website visitors can post or respond to a request for support.

then losing interest once they fade into fashion history. It dissipates with time. Commitment is a cerebral activity, something you work at and focus on because it's important to you, like learning to drive or play a musical instrument.

> *All the good intentions in the world and wishes made on shooting stars have never made anyone thinner.*

When you are up against lifelong eating habits and the mindless comfort of doing things that are familiar, it is not enough to be sincere about losing weight. You must treat it as a serious business.

The first thing you have to do is to complete the *Wedding Dress Diet* 'Weight Loss Contract' on pages 40–41. Once you decide how much weight you can safely lose between today and the wedding (see the *Wedding Dress Diet* 'Worksheet' in Chapter Four), you need to enlist the help of some significant supporters. You can ask your fiancé, your bridesmaids, your mum, your personal trainer, or the whole lot of them if it will help! Each person must be informed of your weight-loss plan and given a specific role to play to help you reach your goal. They, in turn, must be willing to execute their end of the deal by providing the contracted support and enforcing the stated rewards and penalties.

You can use your supporters to do all kinds of things, such as shopping for food for you, cooking a meal for you, washing your gym clothes, or refusing to go to happy hour with you.

A supporter's most important job is witnessing and recording your weigh-ins.

As humbling an experience as this may be, it is also one of the most powerful motivators around. Do yourself a favour, however, by scheduling your weigh-ins for Fridays, not Mondays. People tend to eat more sensibly and exercise more regularly during the weekdays rather than on weekends. A Monday weigh-in can be very discouraging.

Chart your weekly weight on the *Wedding Dress Diet* 'Weight Record' which you'll find in this chapter. We've included both a blank chart for your use and a filled-in sample so that you can see how it works. We've set the chart up for 26 weeks' worth of weight recording. If you have more time than that, be sure to photocopy the blank chart before you begin filling it in.

If you reach your weekly (or monthly) weight-loss goals, you deserve to be rewarded. If you fail to reach them, you must accept a penalty on top of the extra lbs. The rewards and penalties should be meaningful ones to you or they won't motivate you to do what you must, while discouraging you from what you must not!

Money is a major source of motivation for most people. You could set up a system where you put a significant amount of cash into a kitty at the start of your programme – let's say £5 per lb you want to lose. Each week or month that you lose the weight you need to, you can take some of that money back, at a rate of £5 per lb. When you don't lose, that same amount of money must

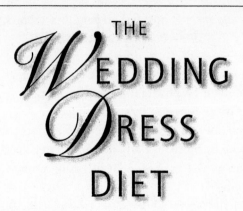

THE WEDDING DRESS DIET

WEIGHT-LOSS CONTRACT

I, _____ , have set the following

specific and measurable weight-loss goal for myself. I pledge

to lose _____ lbs by _____ .

I will follow the dietary guidelines and perform the exercise

outlined in *The Wedding Dress Diet* Worksheet (Chapter 4)

necessary to lose _____ lbs per week/month beginning

on _____ . It is important to me

because _____

_____ .

I have made the following people aware of my goal and they

have agreed to help me achieve it by doing the following

things:

Support Person	Method of Help
1 _____	_____
2 _____	_____
3 _____	_____

I will keep track of my progress by being weighed weekly/monthly. Support Person _____ will witness and enter the results of each weigh-in in *The Wedding Dress Diet Weight Record*. Support Person _____ will serve as the alternate for weigh-ins if the first appointee is unavailable. My reward(s) for losing the required weight at each weigh-in will be _____. My penalty(ies) for not losing the required weight will be _____. A signed and dated copy of this contract has been given to all those named in it.

Bride's signature	_____
Date	_____
Support person 1	_____
Date	_____
Support person 2	_____
Date	_____
Support person 3	_____
Date	_____

be given to someone completely undeserving, such as a lazy teenage sibling or an insufferable colleague who never repays his debts.

You may also arrange for your rewards to be in the form of favours from your supporters. Demand to be pampered with a pedicure or a bedtime backrub for a job well done. Likewise, the penalty for not losing may be that you have to clean your girlfriend's apartment or wash your fiancé's car. Whatever you decide, it has to be meaningful and enforceable to keep you on track. No lame excuses accepted.

After everyone has signed the contract, don't just stuff it into a desk drawer. Keep it out as a visible reminder of the goals you have set for yourself and the hard work that must be done to achieve them. It is helpful to reread your contract once a day to refocus your attention on your goal and strengthen your resolve to see it through to the end.

If you occasionally get off track, or completely lose your way, reach out to your supporters for encouragement. Pick up the phone and call a girlfriend as soon as you feel yourself slipping. Ask her to read the contract aloud to you. Or solicit your signers by e-mail to send you some positive affirmations that you can do it and are going to make it to the wedding in the dress size of your dreams.

Remember, losing weight is hard. If it were easy, everybody would be thin!

Deciding to eat a piece of fruit every afternoon, for example, instead of a vending machine snack sounds simple enough. But to break the old habit, you must put into place several new behaviours.

First, you must have a steady supply of fresh fruit on hand, which means making regular trips to the supermarket. Then you must remember to throw a piece into your bag each morning before you head off to work or to do errands. And then, when you are tired, bored and/or frustrated in the late afternoon, you must resist the temptation to munch on something chocolatey or salty from the vending machine – a path you've walked every day at 3 pm for months – but reach instead into your bag for that piece of fruit!

This is the challenge, but you are as ready now as you will ever be to conquer it. You've got the ring on your finger, the date on the calendar and the dress of your dreams to keep you going. Good luck, and may the best bride lose!

For better and for worse

Before you change the way you eat, you must first change the way you think. Too often, women begin weight-loss programmes when they feel their very worst about themselves. Unfortunately, it only makes the job of losing weight harder if you start off believing you are a hopeless mess.

The Wedding Dress Diet *weight record*

	Weeks	1	2	3	4	5	6	7
	Weigh-in Dates							

Starting Date: _____

Starting Weight: _____

Weight Goal: _____

Goal Date: _____

Weigh-in Weights (lbs)

8 9 10 11 12 13 14 15 16 17 18 19 20 21 22 23 24 25 26

The Wedding Dress Diet *weight record*

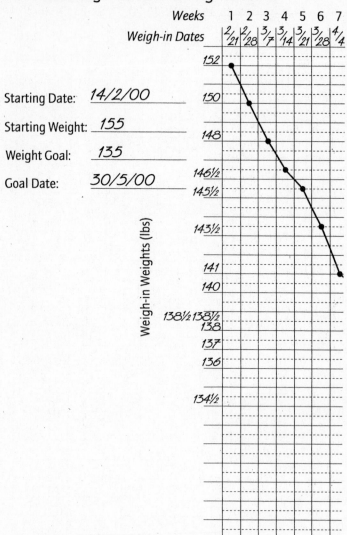

Starting Date: *14/2/00*

Starting Weight: *155*

Weight Goal: *135*

Goal Date: *30/5/00*

9 10 11 12 13 14 15 16 17 18 19 20 21 22 23 24 25 26

$\frac{4}{18}$ $\frac{4}{25}$ $\frac{5}{2}$ $\frac{5}{9}$ $\frac{5}{16}$ $\frac{5}{23}$ $\frac{5}{30}$

Try to imagine lending a helping hand to someone you really don't like. Are you going to go out of your way to make sure she has what she wants? Will you put her needs before your own? Is it likely you'll make personal sacrifices to see that she is happy? Probably not.

Yet if you begin a weight-loss and fitness programme harbouring terrible, negative feelings about yourself, it's the same thing. You are going to need unconditional love and plenty of nurturing to get through the rough times. It isn't possible to provide that if you think yourself unworthy of special care and attention.

Robyn will never forget a former client who really struggled to get her weight down. She rose early each morning to exercise before work and kept track of every morsel she put into her mouth. It seemed no matter how 'good' she was, however, she couldn't make that scale budge more than a few ounces a week. But she didn't become discouraged. She never saw herself as a failure at weight loss. Instead, she recognised that she was doing the best she could, and she accepted the results she got. And she was able to do this because she had many other accomplishments she took pride in.

One summer she decided to renovate her basement to make a playroom for her kids. She got some estimates for the job and quickly realised it would be too expensive to hire a builder, so she decided to do it herself! She watched the home improvement shows on television and read some books on carpentry. Then she measured and designed the room and went to the building supply store for the materials. By the end of the summer, she'd created a fantastic new playroom.

That playroom said more about her than those stubborn little lbs on her hips. She was able to accept the slow pace of her weight loss because she saw herself as more than just a number on the scales. She also realised that she could have just as easily gained weight over those months she was only dropping a lb or two if she hadn't held fast to her programme.

What is important to remember is that having a few lbs or inches to lose does not make you a criminal.

In fact, it doesn't even make you a petty offender. Your moral character cannot be judged by your body weight at all. Focusing all of your attention on a single trait, such as 20 extra lbs, can really undermine your self-confidence, which will, in turn, sabotage your efforts to lose that weight.

It is time to look at all of your attributes so you can see those 10, 20, 30 or 50 extra lbs as a minor flaw when stacked against all your other fine qualities. Once you learn to like yourself for the person you are, it will be much easier to change the packaging you walk around in. You may even come to realise that no improvements are needed after all.

Read the list of features in the chart 'More Than Meets the Eye' on pages 50–51. Check off all that apply to you. Don't be modest. If friends tell you that you have

More than meets the eye

I am able to:

- [ ] Accept criticism
- [ ] Concentrate
- [ ] Control my temper
- [ ] Express my fears
- [ ] Show sympathy
- [ ] Make decisions
- [ ] Meet people
- [ ] _____
- [ ] Take responsibility
- [ ] Organise things
- [ ] Complete projects
- [ ] Make friends
- [ ] Have fun
- [ ] Listen
- [ ] Forgive
- [ ] _____

I have a good:

- [ ] Education
- [ ] Imagination
- [ ] Sense of direction
- [ ] Sense of humour
- [ ] Sense of rhythm
- [ ] Sense of style
- [ ] _____
- [ ] Reputation
- [ ] Memory
- [ ] Personality
- [ ] Religious faith
- [ ] Vocabulary
- [ ] Will-power
- [ ] _____

I am:

- [ ] Articulate
- [ ] Artistic
- [ ] Assertive
- [ ] Athletic
- [ ] Creative
- [ ] Dependable
- [ ] Generous
- [ ] Intelligent
- [ ] Loyal
- [ ] Patient
- [ ] Self-confident
- [ ] Self-disciplined
- [ ] Self-sufficient
- [ ] Sensitive

- ☐ Graceful
- ☐ Happy
- ☐ Hard working
- ☐ Independent
- ☐ _____

- ☐ Sentimental
- ☐ Sexy
- ☐ Thrifty
- ☐ Tolerant
- ☐ _____

Accomplishments in my life I am most proud of:

_____
_____
_____
_____
_____

Talents and/or abilities I possess that others admire in me:

_____
_____
_____
_____
_____

Things about myself I would never want to change:

_____
_____
_____
_____
_____

a great sense of humour, or colleagues marvel at your creativity, then add it to the list! Use the space on the bottom of the chart to list all the personal accomplishments you are most proud of, such as having travelled round the world and your special talents, such as never forgetting anyone's birthday. Then note the things about yourself that you would never want to change.

Use this chart to keep your weight-loss goal in perspective and to stop the flood of negative thoughts that can fill your mind when you've had a minor setback. No one is perfect. And those who think they are already have at least one thing against them!

CHAPTER THREE

Finding the Perfect Wedding Dress for Your Figure

Yes, we know that this chapter seems too premature, coming as it does before the chapters on diet and exercise. But there's a reason: you'll find that you'll have to order your gown a minimum of three months in advance.

*F*or some elaborate dresses, you may have to order up to nine months in advance. Most commonly, the 'lead time' required is about four to six months.

You can understand the problem with this if you haven't yet begun the Wedding Dress Diet and your wedding is, say, four months away. You're apt to be several lbs lighter on the day of your last fitting than you were on the day you ordered the dress. This is why it's important that you also build in at least two weeks for alterations. And take solace from this: it's much easier to take a seam in than it is to take one out!

In perpetuity

The Greek philosopher Heraclitus once said, 'There is nothing permanent except change.' We beg to differ with his eminence.

> *Your basic body structure*
> *is permanent too.*

We'll forgive Heraclitus, however, because he made his statement around 500 BC and women back then were no doubt far more preoccupied with simply surviving each

---

day than they were with figuring out whether they were apple-or pear-shaped. However, the fact is that even if you reach your goal weight on *The Wedding Dress Diet*, your basic body structure will remain the same. In other words, if your hip measurement is significantly larger than your bust size, you'll still be a pear . . . albeit a thin pear. And you'll still look better in some styles than you will in those designed to complement your opposite type: the woman who is bigger on top than on the bottom.

We think 'pear or apple?' is far too broad a generalisation, however. We much prefer the 'H-O-A-X' system of body type classification. Not long ago, Jacqueline had the pleasure of interviewing the woman who developed the H-O-A-X system, Mary Duffy, long employed by the Ford Model Agency in New York City. Basically, each letter – H, O, A and X – visually represents a body type. An 'X' structure, for example, describes a woman with an hourglass figure, a woman whose bust and hip measurements are almost identical, while her waist measurement is significantly smaller.

We're going to use the H-O-A-X system, the apple versus pear division, plus many more specific classifications in the next several pages to help you choose a gown that will both maximise your assets and minimise those you're not so proud of. Circle all the descriptions that apply to you and make notes to take along on your shopping forays. Besides your style preferences, the bridal consultant will want to know your budget, your wedding date and the relative formality of your ceremony.

First, however, here's a glossary of the wedding apparel terms we'll be using. Keep in mind that these aren't the only styles you'll run into in the bridal shop, they're just the ones we suggest in the pages to come.

Glossary of style terms

Silhouette Styles

A-line – Resembles the letter A in that it hugs the body at the shoulders and then flares gradually away from the bodice to the hem. It doesn't have a distinct waistline.

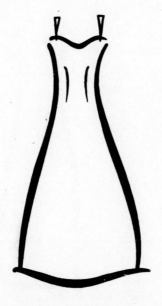

Ballgown – Often paired with a fitted bodice, this gown has a full skirt.

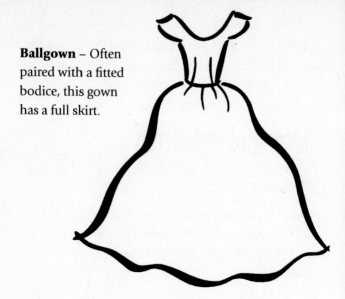

Empire – A high waistline with a seam just under the bustline.

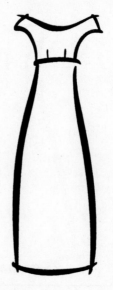

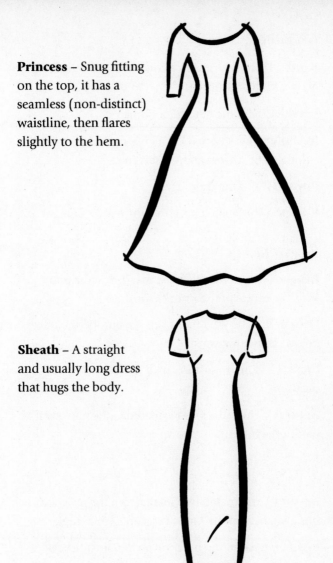

Princess – Snug fitting on the top, it has a seamless (non-distinct) waistline, then flares slightly to the hem.

Sheath – A straight and usually long dress that hugs the body.

Necklines

Band – This neckline has a collar that encircles the neck, a bit like a mock turtleneck.

Jewel – Circles the natural neckline.

Keyhole yoke – Generally, a high-necked dress with cutouts at the throat and/or bustline.

Portrait – Off the shoulders.

V-neck – This angled neckline forms a V shape.

Waistlines

Basque – An elongated waist that drops to a point, or V, in the centre of the front of the dress.

Dropped – The waistline seam is a number of inches below the natural waist.

Empire – A high waistline with a seam just under the bustline.

Natural – The waist seam is placed at the narrowest part of the midriff.

Skirts

Apron – Extra material that falls from the waist much like a kitchen apron. Gives the skirt a fuller look.

Bustle – A gathering of fabric on the outside back of the skirt – sometimes enhanced with no-show padding – to puff out the skirt and make for a 'perkier' bottom.

Flounced or tiered – A skirt with many layers.

Peplum – A flounce or short, flared flap attached at the waist of the dress and puffing out at the hips to enhance, or create, an hourglass figure.

Sleeves

Cap sleeves – Just barely cover the shoulders; short and fitted.

Headpieces

Juliet cap – This small hat hugs the back of the head.

Pillbox – Made famous by Jackie Onassis in the 1960s, this is a round, brimless hat that sits on top of the head.

Tiara – A crown resplendent with pearls, rhinestones, crystals, or other dazzling gems (faux or not).

Veils

Ballet or waltz length – Reaches to the ankles or floor.

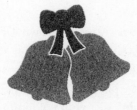

Maximise/minimise with your dress and accessories

Tick all the assets/liabilities that apply. Take notes and then go shopping.

☐ **'I have a small waist'**
Emphasise it with a fitted bodice and a natural or princess waistline.

☐ **'My waist is too thick'**
Team a higher-waisted bodice (such as an empire style) with an A-line skirt.

☐ **'I'm short-waisted'**
Balance yourself with a basque, dropped, or other low waistline (except if you're short in height, as well).

☐ **'I'm a little buxom'**
Show off your voluptuousness with a strapless gown, or one with a portrait or deep V neckline or a keyhole yoke.

☐ **'I'm too buxom'**
You want to draw the eye down. Do so with an elongated bodice (such as basque style) and a full skirt. Treat empire-waisted dresses like the plague; styles that are pinched in at the natural waistline will also emphasise your voluptuousness. Avoid

frills on the bodice, a low neckline and puffy
sleeves. Go for lace or detailing on the skirt's
hemline.

☐ 'I have a long, graceful neck'
Keep your eye out for dresses with a band neckline
or a high-necked keyhole yoke.

☐ 'My neck is too skinny'
Necklaces and chokers are great disguises.

☐ 'I have long, shapely legs'
Search for a short dress or a long sheath that's split
to the thigh.

☐ 'My legs are heavy'
If you're wearing a short dress – though a long
dress might be better for you – opt for sheer or
opaque stockings. Avoid stockings with heavy
textures. Avoid shoes with ankle straps. Look for a
chunky heel; skinny heels on your shoes will also
call attention to the heaviness of your legs.

☐ 'My legs are too skinny'
If you're wearing a short dress, you're the person
who can benefit from heavy-textured stockings. If
your dress reveals your legs, make sure it's not so
full as to make your legs look like straws.

☐ 'I have shapely arms'
Sleeveless dresses, those with cap sleeves and those
with portrait necklines are all good choices.

☐ **'My arms are too plump'**
Opt for long, thin, but not skintight, sleeves.

☐ **'My arms are too skinny'**
Again, go for long sleeves that are not skintight.

☐ **'I have gorgeous hands and nails'**
Attract the eye to them with long sleeves that taper
to a point on the back of your hand.

☐ **'I have bony shoulders/a protruding collarbone'**
Detract from them with a high neckline. Avoid
clingy fabrics (such as jersey) and big puffed
sleeves; the latter will make you look like you're
drowning!

☐ **'I have broad shoulders'**
'Narrow' them with a draped, wide-collared or V
neckline. Avoid shoulder pads and puffed sleeves,
as well as halter dresses and deeply scooped
necklines.

☐ **'I have small hips'**
You can beautifully pull off wearing a gown with a
bustle, peplum and/or apron.

☐ **'I am tall and slim'**
Choose a ballgown-type wedding dress or a long,
narrow sheath.

☐ **'I'm short and chubby'**
Opt for a high waistline such as the empire, a
blousy bodice and long, narrow (but not

skintight) sleeves. Choose a gathered waist
(especially the basque) to make you appear taller.
Stay away from puffy and/or flounced skirts.
Choose a Juliet cap for your headpiece.

☐ *'I'm short, average and want to look taller'*
A high waistline (like the empire) will give the
illusion of more height, but so, on the other hand,
will the deep V of a basque waistline. Avoid full
skirts and full trains . . . a chapel-length train is
right for you. So is a ballet- or waltz-length veil
that skims the body rather than billowing around
it. Other ways to add 'height': choose a high
neckline and short, straight sleeves or, if your arms
are good, go sleeveless with long gloves. If you
choose a short dress, wear pumps rather than
shoes with ankle straps, which tend to make you
look shorter by cutting off your feet at the ankle.
Buy stockings similar if not identical in colour to
your dress; this will give the impression of a longer
line. Your headpiece of choice: the Juliet cap.

☐ *'I'm overweight'* (no matter what your height)
Be on the lookout for gowns with vertical lines,
such as those provided by high-neckline styles that
just skim the body (the princess cut or an empire
waist with an A-line skirt). Another way to create
vertical lines is to wear a long strand of pearls or
beads. No puffed sleeves! And don't buy a dress in a
clingy or thick (such as velvet) fabric. When you go
to choose a headpiece, lean towards a Juliet cap.

☐ **'My feet are too big'**
Opt for a pump with a squared-off or rounded toe
or go with an open-toed shoe. Shoes with pointed
toes, especially those with sling backs, make feet
look even longer than they are.

☐ **'I have a round, full face'**
You can add height with a tiara or pillbox hat. For
your dress, opt for vertical lines. Choose a V-neck
over a rounded, scoop neckline.

☐ **'I have a long, narrow face'**
If you're hoping to achieve a serene, old-fashioned
look, add width with a wide-brimmed hat.
Otherwise, you can add width to your face by
wearing a light-coloured headband or a tiara that
is low and broad.

☐ **'I wear glasses'**
A tiara will be especially flattering.

H-O-A-X hints

These are drawn from Mary Duffy's H-O-A-X system of
classifying body types. See the beginning of this chapter
for more information.

'H' This is the ladder-like figure; one that's straight
up and down with no curves. Create curves by
selecting a style that emphasises both your bustline and
your hips, preferably one that's equal in both areas.

What will help: oversize shoulders, a jewel neckline, a cinched, natural waistline and a full, billowing skirt. Avoid narrow sheaths and empire and other high-waisted styles. They'll add to your 'H-ness'.

'O' The woman with this figure type tends to look round; she carries most of her excess weight in her midriff area. This kind of body is also often accompanied by relatively slender legs so play them up with a short dress or a longer one that's slit up the side. Give yourself a more 'hourglass' appearance by looking for a dress that has an indented (but not fitted) waist and a blousy-style bodice. A V neckline is also a good choice for you.

'A' The pear-shaped figure. Go for styles that are narrow above the waist and wide below. A princess-line gown will narrow your shape while still showing off your feminine curves. Opt for full sleeves that make your shoulders look broader; a high neckline is a no-no because it will make your shoulders look narrower, emphasising your pear-like silhouette. Also avoid narrow, sheathlike styles.

'X' The hourglass body type. You meet the qualifications if your bust and hip measurements are the same and your waist is about 10 inches (25 cm) smaller. Choose a ballgown look: low neckline, off-the-shoulder sleeves, a narrow waistline and a full skirt. Pass up high-waisted styles – they hide all of your assets!

Make-up that maximises/ minimises

Here's the basic principle: Light maximises, dark minimises. Use highlights (the 'light') and contours (the 'dark') to play up or play down your features. You can purchase products especially designed for highlighting or contouring. Or, for highlighting, use a slightly lighter shade of foundation than the one you wear on the rest of your face; lighter-toned cover stick, cream, or liquid; or translucent or pearlised powder. For contouring, you can also try a foundation in a slightly darker shade than you wear on the rest of your face or a gel or powder blusher. The following tips are for that 'extra-special' look you'll want on your wedding day; they're probably a bit over the top for everyday wear.

☐ *'My face is too round'*
Contour with inverted triangles of blusher that start on your cheekbones, stretch under the outer two-thirds of your eyes, and that are well-blended up and out towards your ears and the outer corners of your eyes. Do keep in mind that a bottom-heavy or round face never kept Andie MacDowell or Minnie Driver from getting plum movie roles.

☐ *'My cheeks are too fat'*
Concentrate your blusher or other contour away
from the centre of your face. Sweep it on the sides
of your face from the lower lip line to just about
an inch or two above your eyebrow.

☐ *'My face is too long and thin'*
Use a contourer on the upper third of your
forehead. Also, put a rectangle of blusher along
the tops of your cheekbones, starting at a point
below the outer third of the eye and blending up
and outward all the way out to the ear, then up
along the hairline until it's just a bit higher than
the eyebrows.

☐ *'My cheekbones are too high'*
Concentrate your contour (blusher in this case) on
the centre of your face, closer to your nose.

☐ *'I have a double chin'*
'Firm' yourself up by applying contour under the
chin (but no lower than the first extra chin) from
behind the earlobe, circling around the underside
of the jawbone and crossing beneath the natural
chinbone.

☐ *'My neck is too short'*
Apply contour (in this case, blusher would probably work best) down the sides of the neck,
blending well. This will give the illusion of a
longer neck.

Hairstyles that help

☐ **'I have a round face'**
Do avoid slicked-back and very short hair. A few face-framing curls are in order, as is a side parting.

☐ **'My cheeks are too fat'**
Choose a style that will give you softness and height at the crown and that will keep your hair close to your head on the sides. The latter will give your cheeks the 'shadows' they're missing.

☐ **'My face is too long and thin'**
You want fullness and softness on the sides of your head. A straight fringe will also help.

☐ **'My neck is too fat'**
Opt for a style that's short and simple and keep your hair clear of your neckline.

Know before you go (shopping)

♥ Look behind you. Pay attention to the way the dress looks from behind. That's the way your guests will be seeing you at least half the time.

♥ Most bridal shops require a deposit when you place your order. Often, if you cancel, you'll not only forfeit that deposit, you'll have to pay for the rest of the dress as well. Ask about the shop's cancellation policy *before* you place your order.

❤ Welcome to your new, bigger size. Most wedding dresses run small, at least a size or two, and you'll find this to be especially true if you're busty or broad-shouldered. At any rate, don't faint at the bridal consultant's announcement that you need, say, a size 16 instead of your regular size 12.

❤ But you'll probably feel pretty small in another way . . . and that's in terms of length. Most gowns are made to fit a woman who is 5ft 8in. Hemming may be on your horizon.

❤ Dress to impress. When you go for fittings, wear undergarments and accessories that are similar or the same as the ones you plan to wear on your wedding day, such as a push-up Wonderbra, light stockings and high heels.

❤ Home shopping. Besides studying the bridal magazines, you can get lots of ideas from the hundreds of Websites devoted to wedding dresses. Just type the key words 'wedding dresses' or 'wedding gowns' into your search engines. One website we particularly like is www.Wedding Channel.com. There's a page on this Website that will show you gowns based on your preferences in silhouette, waistline, length, neckline, sleeve length, sleeve style, fabric type, skirt style, train style and colour.

Picture perfect

Of course you'll want to show off your new look – and your new dress – to best advantage in your wedding photos. We got the following tips from professional photographer Stephen Trobaugh.

While standing for a photo: place your feet slightly apart in a modified T position – that is, with your 'leading' foot pointing straight at the camera and the other foot behind it and nearly perpendicular to the heel of the lead foot. Put your weight on the back foot and slightly bend your front knee. Put your shoulders back and turn the upper part of your body towards the camera. This position is halfway between a profile and a straight-on shot and makes for the best silhouette. A straight-on shot would emphasise any 'hippiness'; a profile would do the same for a problem tummy or butt.

If you're not holding flowers, lightly rest your leading hand on your thigh. Your other arm can be slightly behind your back or down the side of the corresponding thigh.

When sitting: again, your body should not be faced directly at the camera. Sit on the edge of the chair (slight camera lens distortion is exaggerated when you lean away from the camera; it can make you look 'slouchy'). Sit up straight, knees together, one foot in front of the other. For a graceful look, clasp your hands and place them on top of one leg or the other – not in the middle. Same goes for flowers.

About spectacles: if you'll be wearing them in your pictures, you'll have to lower your chin a bit so that the camera flash won't hit the middle of your glasses, obscuring your eyes. If a slight downward tilt of your head would make for, or emphasise, a double chin, you can also prevent flash glare by sliding your glasses down your nose a bit.

If you regularly wear glasses but will not be wearing them in your photos, be sure to take them off about 15 minutes in advance so that your red 'nose marks' will have faded, or use a concealer.

About undergarments: Stephen Trobaugh told us that the problem he encounters most often in wedding photography, surprisingly, is that someone's bra strap or even the top of her bra is showing. Pin judiciously! And assign a woman who is not in the wedding party to be especially alert for this problem during every posed photograph.

Another undergarment problem Trobaugh has faced is that a bridesmaid's dress or even the bride's gown is so sheer that lingerie shows through in flash pictures. You might want to keep this in mind when you shop for your wedding finery!

About background: let's say you and your bridesmaids are having your pre-wedding pictures taken at your mum's house. Her flowered wallpaper, striped drapes and photo-covered panelled walls have been around so long that you don't really 'see' them any more. Well, that'll change when you get your wedding photos back and those backgrounds are 'busy' or they clash horribly with your bridesmaids' dresses. Try to see potential backgrounds as if you are looking through the eyes of a stranger, and opt for a setting that's colour complementary or undistracting. A fireplace is a good example of the latter.

About crying: you're bound to do some crying and a lot of kissing on your big day. Before every picture, ask your maid of honour if you need to touch up your lipstick or wipe off a smudge of mascara.

Put together a fix-it kit:

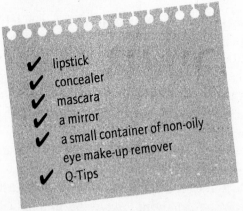

- ✔ lipstick
- ✔ concealer
- ✔ mascara
- ✔ a mirror
- ✔ a small container of non-oily eye make-up remover
- ✔ Q-Tips

Carry the kit in one of those satin bridal pouch purses you wear dangling from your wrist. One enterprising bride we know even had a pocket sewn into her wedding gown in which to keep her fix-its. This may be an option for you if the skirt of your dress is full.

CHAPTER FOUR

The Calorie Count- down

Diets come and diets go, but calories are forever. No matter how clever the latest weight-loss gimmick of the month might sound, it all boils down to the calories at the weigh-in.

*Y*our *Wedding Dress Diet* is anchored by the number of calories you eat each day and the amount of vigorous activity you perform each week. There are several different ways to space the timing of your meals and combine the foods you eat at them. This will not affect how fast or how much weight you lose.

What kind of foods those calories come from does matter, however, and we need to deal with this first before we talk about calorie counting.

Adult humans simply don't need that much protein or fat to maintain a healthy body or to prevent disease.

Excess fat in the diet can clog the arteries and increases cancer risk, even if you manage to keep your weight under control. Excess protein taxes the kidneys and depletes calcium from the skeleton and that's something most women can't afford to lose. On the other hand, we need a good source of fuel 24 hours a day. Carbohydrates are the best possible form of fuel for humans. Ideally, you should get a small number of your daily calories from fat (such as oil, soft margarine, or butter), a moderate amount from protein (such as lean meats, poultry and fish) and the greatest amount from carbohydrates (such as bread, cereals, fruits and many vegetables). In percentages, this means you should get 20 per cent of your total calories from fat, 25 per cent from protein, and the remaining 55 per cent from carbohydrates. You can use the chart below to determine the number of grams of fat, protein and carbohydrate recommended for different calorie levels based on these percentages.

Distributing your calories

Calories	Fat grams	Protein grams	Carbohydrate grams
1,200	27	75	165
1,300	29	80	180
1,400	31	87	193
1,500	33	94	206
1,600	35	100	220
1,700	38	106	234
1,800	40	112	248
1,900	42	119	261
2,000	44	125	275

Nutrition basics

The simplest and most reliable way to ensure that your diet is nutritionally sound is to eat for colour, texture and calcium.

For **Colour**, choose at least three servings of fruit each day and three vegetables in shades of red, orange, green and yellow (see the chart below) (sample serving sizes provided on pages 100–1). The produce aisle is packed with the vitamins, minerals and phytochemicals (cancer fighters) that will keep your hair, skin and nails glowing and your immune system strong. You can vary your selections with the seasons and enjoy your produce fresh, frozen without sugar, canned in natural juice, dried, or as 100 per cent juice to meet your quota. In the case of the latter, however, don't 'drink' all of your fruits and vegetables. Yes, such juices are chock-full of the same vitamins and phytochemicals as solid produce, but they don't pack the fibre . . . or the chewing satisfaction!

Colour schemes for good health

Red	Orange	Green	Yellow
Apple	Apricot	Asparagus	Banana
Beets	Cantaloupe	Bok choy	Cassava
Cherries	Carrot	Broccoli	Corn
Plum	Mango	Collard greens	Grapefruit
Raspberries	Orange juice	Grapes	Lemon
Red cabbage	Peach	Figs	Onion
Salsa	Pumpkin	Honeydew	Papaya
Strawberries	Tangerine	Pear	Pineapple
Sweet pepper	Squash	Peas	Turnips
Tomato	Yam	Spinach	Pepper

(Be sure to thoroughly wash your fruits and vegetables before eating or cooking.)

Texture comes from chewy wholegrains and cereals and the stone-ground flours and meals made from them. Because wholegrains still have their outer bran layer intact, they are higher in fibre than their white, refined counterparts. Fibre fills us up without filling us out. These grains are also high in complex carbohydrates, the kind that supply a steady source of energy for hours after eating them. Choose at least three servings a day of the following wholesome, high-fibre, high-energy foods to keep you going all day, and all night, if necessary.

Calcium is a critical nutrient for women of all ages, not just little girls. If you have been careless about your

The taste of texture

Wholegrains	Cereals	Flour and meal products
Brown rice	Bran flakes	Bran muffin
Barley	Wheat flakes	Corn bread
Buckwheat	Rice flakes	Polenta
Bulgur	Corn flakes	Popcorn
Cracked wheat	Muesli	Ryvita crackers
Quinoa	Oatmeal	Soba noodles
Rye	Puffed rice	Taboule
Wild rice	Shredded wheat	Tortilla
Wheat berries	Wheatgerm	Wholewheat pasta

intake of calcium-rich dairy products up to now, it is time to take your bones seriously before they leave you slouching. During your childbearing years, you need at least three servings a day of high-calcium foods (300 mgs per serving – see page 82). If you can't or you won't or you don't eat at least three good sources of calcium every day, buy a supplement today and take 1,000 mgs a day until age 50. Then you can increase the dose to 1,500 mgs a day for the rest of your life.

The recommended daily servings of these basic foods will supply approximately 800 calories. You should also have at least one good source of protein. Once these nutrient requirements are met, you are free to fill in the rest of your calorie 'budget' with an eating plan to match your personal schedule and food preferences. But always remember that no weight-loss programme can succeed without your paying strict attention to calories in and energy out.

Working out your workout

Vigorous, aerobic exercise is necessary to use up the calories you have stored in your body as fat. There is a difference between this type of exercise and that done to improve general fitness, such as a daily walk. You have to work off those lbs accumulated at past meals and snacks. This can't be done by taking a stroll in the park. In fact, we're not even talking 'walk' here.

Calcium-to-calories connection

Calcium source	Serving size	Calcium	Calories
Fat-free milk	8 fl oz (250 ml)	300	85
Skimmed milk	8 fl oz (250 ml)	300	100
Whole milk	8 fl oz (250 ml)	300	150
Powdered non-fat milk	2 fl oz (50 ml)	373	110
Fortified low-fat milk	8 fl oz (250 ml)	500	100
Soy milk, fortified	8 fl oz (250 ml)	300	120
Rice milk, fortified	8 fl oz (250 ml)	300	100
Orange juice, fortified	8 fl oz (250 ml)	350	110
Yogurt, low-fat and sweetened	8 fl oz (250 ml)	300	250
Yogurt, low-fat, plain	8 fl oz (250 ml)	400	130
Yogurt, frozen, fat-free with added calcium	4 oz (120 ml)	450	90
Evaporated whole milk	4 fl oz (120 ml)	330	170
Cottage cheese, low-fat with added calcium	4 oz (120 ml)	200	80
Ricotta cheese, fat-free	4 oz (120 ml)	270	100
Cocoa, sugar-free and fortified	1 packet	300	50
Cereal bar, fortified	1 bar	200	130
Soy cheese, fortified	1 oz (25 g)	200	75

Think speed walking, or jogging, or running if you want to get that weight off.

Aerobic exercise can be measured by your heart rate during the workout, not by how much you have perspired or how long you've been exercising. When completing your *Wedding Dress Diet* 'Worksheet' (see page 88), use the chart below to find the exercise heart rate you need to achieve. An explanation of how to measure your exercise heart rate – and also how to calculate your level if you're over 40 years old – can be found in Chapter Five on page 118.

Exercise heart rates

Age	Start-up rate (55% max.)	Intermediate rate (65% max.)	Experienced rate (75% max.)
18	111	131	151
20	110	130	150
22	109	129	149
24	108	127	147
26	107	126	146
28	106	125	144
30	105	124	143
32	103	122	141
34	102	121	140
36	101	120	138
40	99	117	135

Once you know what your exercise heart rate is and how to measure it, you must choose a type of exercise that raises your heart rate to your target level, and you must be able to sustain that activity for 30 minutes or more. How long and how often you work out at your exercise heart rate will determine how fast and how much weight you will ultimately lose.

Resistance exercises, such as weight lifting, are discussed in Chapter Five. They help to increase the amount of muscle in your body, which raises your metabolism and aids weight loss. Resistance exercises are also used to tone and shape the muscles and have also been shown to increase bone density.

Calculating your caloric allowance

Follow these three steps to complete the *Wedding Dress Diet* 'Worksheet' on page 88.

Step 1 – Use the BMI chart on pages 22–3 to determine the high and low weight range for your height. This is generally the weight that falls between a BMI of 20 and 24. The weight range for each height allows for differences in frame size and body composition. Your weight goal should fall within this range. If it doesn't, you may be aiming too low or too high. If you are extremely muscular, you may have to accept a higher weight since muscle weighs more than fat.

Once you have established a healthy goal weight, subtract that number from your present weight. Next, count how many full weeks you have left until the wedding. A weight loss of 1 to 2 lbs a week is what you can safely and comfortably expect.

Now divide the number of lbs you want to lose by the number of weeks until the wedding. If the number is greater than 2 – that is, more than 2 lbs per week of weight loss – you will have to readjust your goal to a higher weight or accept a much stricter limit on caloric intake while increasing your energy output, as outlined in Step 3.

Step 2 – Multiply your goal weight by the activity factor below that matches your time commitment to exercise. The times given are for total hours per week of vigorous aerobic exercise performed at your exercise heart rate. Two hours of a vigorous recreational sport, such as soccer, squash or basketball, can replace one hour of aerobic exercise.

Activity factors

Total exercise per week	Activity factor
Maximum output: 6–7 hours	16
Outstanding output: 5–6 hours	14
Exemplary output: 4–5 hours	13
Acceptable output: 3–4 hours	12
Notable output: 2–3 hours	11
Better than nothing: 1–2 hours	10

Since all good intentions can be undermined by natural disasters, procrastination and lack of time, you need a back-up plan. Calculate at least three levels of caloric intake for yourself based on three different exercise goals. One can be the greatest number of hours a week you can conceivably work out, another the more realistic number of hours you're likely to work out and the third the least number of hours a week you will ever let yourself squeak by with.

With these numbers in hand, you can adjust your daily caloric intake to match your output as the weeks pass. If you don't make the adjustment and continue to eat as if you were exercising five hours a week when, in fact, you've only done three hours, you are not going to lose the weight you need to.

If you exceed your daily calorie allowance only once in a while, you can make up for the excess eating by increasing your output in that week. Every 200 extra calories you eat require another thirty minutes of exercise.

Step 3 (optional) – If your calculations in Step 1 indicate you need to lose 2/3 lbs per week, and you don't want to settle for a higher weight goal, you must make additional adjustments to your plan. First, you must add one more hour of exercise to your weekly workouts, even if you based your calculations on the maximum range of six to seven hours per week. You must also subtract 200 calories from your daily allowance. But pay close attention to the calories-for-height restrictions below. If you hit the lowest calorie level recommended for your height, don't go any lower. You will only slow down your weight loss if your caloric intake is insufficient to meet your basic needs. Why frustrate yourself? Work on styling ideas instead.

Calories-for-height restrictions

Height	Lowest caloric intake
4' 11"–5' 1"	1,000
5' 2"–5' 4"	1,200
5' 5"–5' 7"	1,400
5' 8"–5' 10"	1,600

Keeping tabs on yourself

You now know the caloric 'budget' you must live on to shed those unwanted lbs in time for your walk down the aisle. The next thing you need is a way to stick to that budget.

If you happen to be good at managing your chequebook, you should have no difficulty managing your caloric budget. Actually, it requires the same skills. You write down a lot of numbers, then do some simple addition and subtraction. If you're not really good at money management, this diet will certainly help you get better at it. Just think, you might actually lose weight and save some money at the same time!

The Wedding Dress Diet *worksheet*

(attach to Contract prepared and signed in Chapter 2)

Step 1

Weight range for height, according to BMI: _____ to _____ lbs
low   high

Goal weight: _____ lbs

Present weight: _____ lbs

Weight to be lost: _____ lbs

Weeks until wedding: _____

Weight loss per week _____ ÷ _____ = _____
to reach goal: lbs to lose   weeks   lbs/week

Step 2

Weight Goal	×	Activity Factor	=	Calories Per Day	
_____	×	_____	=	_____	greatest exercise time
_____	×	_____	=	_____	reasonable exercise time
_____	×	_____	=	_____	least exercise time

Step 3 (if trying to lose 2–3 lbs per week)

_____ −200 calories = _____
initial calories   adjusted calories

Planned hours _____ + 1 additional = _____
exercise per week   hour

Here's how it works. When you go shopping or pay your bills, you record the exact amount for each cheque written so you can see that your balance covers your expenses. When trying to lose weight, you must write down the caloric value for everything you eat to be sure you're not going over your daily caloric allowance.

Typically, this is where the groaning and moaning begins. But there is no point in complaining about record keeping. No one can accurately keep track of everything she eats without writing it down. If you were so good at keeping track of what you ate in the first place, you would be thin already!

Research has shown that the people most successful at losing weight and keeping it off are the ones who kept the best food logs. Other studies have demonstrated that when overweight people are interviewed about what they eat, they often under-report their intake by as much as 20 per cent. That can add up to a lot of unreported calories.

Don't despair!

If you do a really good job at keeping your food records for the first two weeks, it becomes much easier after that. You will start to remember the values for the foods you eat regularly and can refer back to former records for items eaten only occasionally.

Some people get frustrated when they can't find an exact calorie value for each and every morsel they eat, so they give up and stop recording anything at all. If you're one of these people, lighten up! The world isn't perfect and some things just aren't knowable. But you can make an educated guess and move on. The worst thing you can do is give yourself an excuse to eat whatever you want when you decide not to keep tabs on yourself any more. An extra thousand calories can be downed in less time than it takes to say 'Häagen-Dazs.'

Working out the caloric (or fat or sodium) values on packaged foods is usually quite simple since all the information you need can generally be found on the Nutrition Facts panel. Just remember to check the serving size specified. If you eat more or less than that amount, you must adjust your nutritional calculations accordingly.

*Bear in mind that the serving sizes
listed by some manufacturers
are absurdly small.*

If you don't have a food label to help you, use a calorie guide available in any bookstore or online bookseller. These guides contain the nutritional information for foods without labels, such as fresh fruits, vegetables and meats. They also contain the values for most brand-name packaged foods and many chain restaurant menu items. Be sure to get a guide with a current copyright date since the ingredients in commercial food products often change.

Count, measure and weigh each and every day

Once you have your own pocket calorie guide, you can work out the values for everything you put in your mouth – and that's just what you must be willing to do. No exceptions. Every Polo, broken biscuit, stray chip and swig of your fiancé's beer must be duly recorded and added to your total.

What you will quickly realise, as every veteran calorie counter has before you, is that calories are tied to quantities. This is the line that divides the losers and the gainers. If you aren't prepared to take control of how much you really eat, as opposed to the amount you think you ate, or guess you ate, or estimate you ate, you may be off by hundreds of calories a day!

Without question, ladies, it is portion control that separates the size 10s from the size 20s.

Another food fact you'll no doubt pick up on is that anything high in fat is also high in calories. If you want to make those precious calories last longer, steer clear of very high-fat foods. This means anything deep fried, most processed meats, mince, full-fat cheeses and, of course, cakes, biscuits and desserts

But keep in mind, too, that no food is forbidden. Whatever your taste buds demand can be put into your budget – just don't get carried away or you won't be able to squeeze into that wedding gown.

What you must be prepared to do is juggle your calories to make some of the higher-fat food choices fit. Fortunately, there are plenty of very low-fat and low-calorie fruits and vegetables to fill up on the rest of the day after you eat that high-fat, high-calorie hot dog at the cinema.

So how will you go about mastering your portion control? You can start by buying a set of food scales, a set of US measuring cups if you can get them, and a set of measuring spoons. Then you must spend a week checking the capacity of every drinking glass, coffee mug, cereal bowl, dessert dish, wineglass, soup ladle etc in your household. Once you know how much each of these utensils holds, you won't have to remeasure every food and drink you consume from them.

Making careful observations of the serving sizes for foods you prepare or eat at home will also help train your eye for those occasions when you are eating out and cannot weigh and measure your food. Even then, there are ways to make accurate estimates. For some helpful guidelines, see the Relative Food Portions section on pages 100–2.

Armed with these record-keeping tools, you are now ready to start writing. You'll find the *Wedding Dress Diet* 'Food and Fitness Log' on pages 94–5. You can photocopy the sample page or design a spreadsheet on your computer or write the headings onto the pages of a small notebook. What you choose to use for your log is entirely up to you, as long as it is convenient for you and gets the job done. Following the blank chart, you'll find a sample of a filled-in chart.

Instructions for completing the food and fitness log

Once you have a place to record your food and fitness activities, keep it handy and be ready to write whenever you eat. Start each day by entering the day of the week and the date on the top of a new record. Then:

❤ Note the time you eat or drink something and write it on your log before listing the foods and beverages you consumed.

❤ Record the amount of each item eaten or drunk using actual weight in ounces or grams, or the volume in fluid ounces, litres, or measuring spoons, or the counted number of pieces, or the size in inches or centimetres.

❤ Describe the food using the brand name (such as Special K cereal) or type of food (chicken breast). List each item individually if you have a combination food. For example, your ham and cheese sandwich should be recorded as '2 slices wholemeal bread, 3 oz ham, 1 oz Swiss cheese, 1 tablespoon mustard'.

❤ Note any special features of the foods, such as 'reduced-calorie version', or 'cooked in broth in

The Wedding Dress Diet food and fitness log

Day _____ Date _____

Time	Amount	Description of Food	Special Features	Calories	Fruit/Veg	Grain	Calcium

TOTAL

Aerobic Activity _____ Duration: _____ Exercise Heart Rate: _____

Resistance Exercises: Upper Body: _____ Lower Body: _____ Abs: _____

Supplements: ☐ Yes ☐ No Goals Reached: ☐ Yes ☐ No

If not, what will you do differently tomorrow? _____

The Wedding Dress Diet food and fitness log

Day **Saturday**   Date **17 July 1999**

Time	Amount	Description of Food	Special Features	Calories	Fruit/Veg	Grain	Calcium
8.30am	115g	Cottage cheese	1% low fat	90			1
	½	Cantaloupe		75	1		
	50g	Wheatgerm		100		1	
	350ml	Coffee	brewed	0			
	2 tbsp	Milk	1% low fat	15			⅛
10am	15cm	Banana		100	1		
11am	350ml	Water		0			
12.30pm	20cm	Tortilla		85		1¼	
	50g	Turkey breast		80			
	75g	Sprouts		5	½		
	75g	Roasted peppers		5	½		
	50g	Cheddar cheese	grated	100			1

Time	Food	Description		Cal			
	350ml Lemonade	sugar free		0			
2.00pm	180ml Hot chocolate	sugar free, low fat		50		1	
	18g Muesli bar			110			1
5.30pm	8 Baby carrots			40	1		
	2 tbsp French dressing	low fat		50			
6.30pm	175g Cooked brown rice			200	2		
	250g Chinese vegs	stir fry		250	2		
	75g Prawns			85			
	75g Chocolate mousse	low fat		70			¼
	TOTAL			1510	6	5¼	3⅜

Aerobic Activity __Cross Trainer__   Duration: __45 min__   Exercise Heart Rate: __140 bpm__

Resistance Exercises: Upper Body: __Yes__   Lower Body: __Yes__   Abs: __Yes__

Supplements: ☑ Yes ☐ No   Goals Reached: ☐ Yes ☑ No

If not, what will you do differently tomorrow? __Drink more water with meals__ wok', or 'skin removed from chicken', or 'home made recipe' ,or 'fortified with extra calcium'.

- ♥ Look up the caloric value for each item and calculate the actual number of calories in the amount you ate. You may want to subtotal your daily calories after each meal so that you know how many more you have left to work with that day.

- ♥ Indicate if any item is a full or partial serving of your daily requirement for fruits/vegetables, grains or calcium-rich foods and write in the number under the appropriate heading. This will let you know how you're doing nutrition-wise. See 'Standardised Serving Sizes' immediately following this section for examples of standardised portions for these foods.

- ♥ Total your calories at the end of the day. Also total the number of servings of fruits/vegetables, grain and calcium.

- ♥ Enter what type of aerobic exercise you did and for how long, and whether your exercise heart rate was monitored and maintained.

- ♥ Indicate whether you completed your scheduled resistance workout for upper and lower body and abdominal exercises.

- ♥ Tick whether or not you have taken your required supplements.

- ♥ Tick whether or not you achieved your food and fitness goals on this day. If not, state what you will do tomorrow to meet them.

Standardised serving sizes

One serving equals any of the following:

Fruit

★ Any whole piece of fruit the size of a tennis ball
★ 5 oz (125 g) of cubed or balled fresh fruit, whole berries, or grapes
★ 5 oz (125 g) diced fruit, canned fruit in its own juice, or full-strength fruit juice
★ 1½ oz (40 g) dried fruit bits

Vegetables

★ 3 oz (75 g) of raw salad greens
★ 10 oz (250 g) of raw coarsely chopped or sliced vegetables
★ 5 oz (125 g) cooked vegetables, all-vegetable soup, stewed tomatoes, or salsa
★ 8 raw pieces the size of an index finger or chunks the size of cherry tomatoes

Grains

★ 1 oz (25 g) slice of wholegrain bread
★ 3 oz (75 g) cooked rice, couscous or pasta
★ 1 oz (25 g) wholegrain cereal flakes (eg bran flakes)

- ★ 2½ oz (50 g) wheatgerm
- ★ 1 oz (25 g) muesli
- ★ 6 wholegrain crackers

Calcium-Rich Foods

- ★ See the Calcium-to-Calories Connection on page 82 or use an amount that provides 200 to 300 mgs of calcium.

Relative food portions

To help you out when you're eating away from home:

Measuring without a ruler	
First joint of index finger	= ½ teaspoon or 1 inch (2.5 cm)
First joint (or tip) of thumb	= 1 teaspoon
Tight fist	= 8 fl oz (250 ml)
Palm of hand (diameter and thickness)	= 3 ozs (125 g)
Flat hand with closed fingers	= 6 oz (150 g)
Spread fingers, from tip of thumb to tip of little finger	= 9 inches (225 cm)

Size and dimension of familiar objects

Standard paper clip	=	1 1/4 inches (3.1 cm) long
Big paper clip	=	1 7/8 inches (4.7 cm) long
Tennis ball/baseball	=	2 1/2 inches in diameter (6.25 cm) or 8 fl oz (250 ml)

Food and object comparisons

4 standard gaming dice	=	1 oz (25 g) of cheese or meat cubes
3 1/2-inch computer disc	=	1 oz (25 g) slice of cheese
Matchbook	=	1 oz (25 g) of meat or cheese
Ping-Pong ball	=	1 oz (25 g) meatball
Golf ball	=	2 tablespoons peanut butter or cream cheese
3 ice cubes	=	4 oz (100 g) rice or 5 oz (125 g) chopped vegetables
Deck of cards	=	3 oz (75 g) meat, poultry, fish
Cassette tape case	=	3 oz (75 g) meat, poultry, fish
Computer mouse	=	4 oz (100 g) meat, poultry, fish
Bar of soap	=	4 oz (100 g) meat, poultry, fish
300-page paperback book	=	8 oz (200 g) meat, poultry, fish

Kitchen science

Weight conversion

Ounce (oz)	Pound (lb)	Gram (g)
1		25
2		50
3		75
4	1/4	100
6		175
8	1/2	225
16	1	450
	1 1/2	675
	2	900

Liquid measures

1 tablespoon	= 3 teaspoons	= 1/2 fl oz	= 15 ml
2 tablespoons		= 1 fl oz	= 30 ml
4 tablespoons	= 1/4 cup	= 2 fl oz	= 50 ml
5 tablespoons	= 1/3 cup	= 2 1/2 fl oz	= 75 ml
8 tablespoons	= 1/2 cup	= 4 fl oz	= 120 ml
10 tablespoons	= 2/3 cup	= 5 fl oz (1/4 pint)	= 150 ml
12 tablespoons	= 3/4 cup	= 6 fl oz	= 175 ml
16 tablespoons	= 1 cup	= 8 fl oz	= 250 ml

CHAPTER FIVE

Exercising for Results

When most people talk about their 'workout', they are referring to the gym they belong to, or the equipment they use, or the activity they prefer. You rarely hear them describe how much it's like a job, or 'work', but that's exactly what exercise is.

*I*f you think just showing up at a step class qualifies as a 'workout', you're wrong. If you think donning your sneakers and taking a walk in your lunch hour is a 'workout', you're wrong, too.

And if you think you can miss a 'workout' because you stayed out too late last night, you're wrong again.

To lose weight, your exercise regimen, or workout, must be approached with the same seriousness you use to tackle any tough job. It doesn't matter whether you're having fun or feel like doing it. You've got to get results (read: lose weight and sculpt muscles), and that means making every session count.

If you were positioning yourself for a promotion at your job you wouldn't leave anything up to chance, would you? One typo on your CV can cancel out everything you've worked so hard to accomplish. When you want to be noticed and get ahead, you must always be on time and properly prepared. That applies to your workouts, too.

Have a plan of action and work your plan. Know where you started and where you want to end up. If you're doing a routine and don't see the desired loss of inches or pounds after a month, stop doing it and start something else that pays you for your effort.

Now for some startling statistics. You have around 600 muscles in your body, with about 400 of them affecting your physique. It is not possible to grow new muscles once you reach adulthood, any more than it is possible to grow taller. But you can tone, shape and strengthen your muscles. The most fit and firm athlete must continually work her muscles or they will shrink and soften. There is no escaping the demands of a muscle. You must use it or lose it.

More frightening for most of us is the fact that there are anywhere between 25 to 75 billion fat cells in the body! Your genetic make-up determines where those fat cells are located and nothing short of liposuction (which we don't recommend) can remove them. Fortunately, you can control how much fat you store in them. Eating an appropriate number of calories while doing regular, vigorous exercise will shrink those fat cells. But if and when you abandon that winning combination, your fat cells will engorge again.

Pick your passion

In Chapter Four, you selected an activity factor to help you determine how many calories a day you can consume to reach your weight goal. Now you must choose the activity(ies) you will engage in every week to satisfy that time commitment. The activity(ies) will be the aerobic, or calorie-burning, part of your workout.

You must be able to perform each activity for at least 30 minutes and maintain your target heart rate while doing it. Be prepared to change the intensity of your workout if your heart rate is too fast or too slow.

Whatever you do, don't become complacent.

Anything that feels too easy or too comfortable might not be 'work' any more. Switch to something new that you're not so good at to be sure the time you put in produces the desired results.

There is no one value for energy expenditure that applies to everyone who does a particular exercise. The calories used when exercising are directly related to body weight. A heavier person will expend more energy than a lighter one if both are doing the same activity at the same intensity.

The list below shows the number of calories burned by women of different weights when performing each activity for one minute. You need to find the weight closest to yours, then look for the exercise you do, or plan to do. The number that intersects your weight and the exercise activity is the number of calories you use per minute while doing that activity. Multiply it by the number of minutes you do the exercise to see how many calories you used up. To lose weight, you should aim for an aerobic exercise goal of burning the same number of calories in one week as you consume in one day. That means if you are eating 1,600 calories per day, you should select exercises, and enough exercise time, to expend 1,600 calories a week.

Another way you can maximise the amount of fat you burn during each workout is to exercise for as long as possible in each session. This allows your fat cells to release their stored deposits because your short-term body fuels, like glucose, cannot cover the longer work sessions. The longer you work out, the more conditioned your fat cells will become to dumping their stored fat into your bloodstream so it can be used as fuel.

To continue exercising for more than 30 minutes, you need to keep intensity at a moderate level. Again, use your heart rate as a guide to whether you are working too hard (more information about calculating your exercise heart rate can be found in the following activity charts).

Sweat is not a measure of how hard you're working!

It simply means your body's internal temperature is heating up and you are cooling yourself off. Some people – such as most guys – just have an inordinate number of sweat glands and can soak a T-shirt without even trying. Use the clock and your heart rate to evaluate your performance.

If you haven't been exercising regularly and are over the age of 35 with more than 30 pounds to lose, consult your physician before beginning any exercise programme.

Calories used per minute for different activities

Activity	Body weights (in lbs)									
	110	123	139	150	163	176	190	203
Aerobic Dance								
Low intensity/impact	4.5	5.0	5.6	6.1	6.7	7.2	7.7	8.0
High intensity/impact	9.2	10.4	11.5	12.6	13.7	14.8	15.9	17.0
Aqua-running								
W/floatation belt								
48/strides/minute	7.3	8.2	9.0	9.9	10.8	11.7	12.5	13.4
Bench-stepping								
30 step cycle/minute								
6-inch bench	7.1	7.9	8.8	9.7	10.5	11.4	12.2	13.1
12-inch bench	8.5	9.5	10.5	11.5	12.5	13.5	14.5	15.6

Activity	Body weights (in lbs)									
	110	123	139	150	163	176	190	203
Bicycling – road								
10–12 mph	5.3	5.9	6.5	7.1	7.8	8.4	9.0	9.7
14–16 mph	8.8	9.8	10.9	11.9	13.0	14.0	15.1	16.1
Stationary bicycling								
60 rpm – 50 watts	3.4	3.8	4.2	4.6	5.0	5.4	5.9	6.3
60 rpm – 100 watts	5.0	5.6	6.2	6.8	7.4	8.0	8.6	9.2
60 rpm – 150 watts	6.6	7.4	8.2	8.9	9.7	10.5	11.3	12.1
Calisthenics								
Home, general, moderate	3.9	4.4	4.9	5.4	5.8	6.3	6.8	7.2
Vigorous	7.0	7.8	8.7	9.5	10.4	11.2	12.0	12.9
Dance								
Ballroom fast and modern, swing, twist	5.3	5.9	6.5	7.1	7.8	8.4	9.0	9.7

Big band, rock'n'roll	4.2	4.7	5.2	5.7	6.2	6.7	7.2	7.7
Equestrian								
Trotting horseback	5.7	6.4	7.1	7.7	8.4	9.1	9.8	10.5
Galloping	7.0	7.8	8.7	9.5	10.4	11.2	12.0	12.9
Gymnastics								
General	3.5	3.9	4.3	4.8	5.2	5.6	6.0	6.4
Ice skating								
Less than 9 mph	4.8	5.4	6.0	6.5	7.1	7.7	8.3	8.9
More than 9 mph	7.9	8.8	9.8	10.7	11.7	12.6	13.5	14.5
Jazzercise								
Moderate	5.8	6.5	7.2	7.9	8.5	9.2	9.9	10.6
W/ 6 × 8-inch bench, music 120 beats/min	7.7	8.6	9.5	10.4	11.3	12.3	13.2	14.1
Kickboxing	8.8	9.9	11.0	12.0	13.1	14.1	15.2	16.3

Activity	Body weights (in lbs)									
	110	123	139	150	163	176	190	203
Mini trampoline								
120 foot strikes/min								
No arm pumping, weights or jumping	6.9	7.7	8.5	9.4	10.2	11.0	11.8	12.7
Arms pumping, holding 1 lb hand weights, 2 foot jumping	8.7	9.7	10.8	11.8	12.9	13.9	15.0	16.0
Roller skating								
Inside, rink	5.7	6.4	7.1	7.7	8.4	9.1	10.1	10.8
Outside, pavement	6.2	7.0	7.7	8.4	9.2	9.9	10.7	11.4
Rollerblading								
Casual	6.7	7.4	8.2	9.0	9.8	10.6	11.4	12.2
Vigorous (12.4 mph on asphalt)	10.6	11.9	13.1	14.4	15.7	16.9	18.2	19.5

Rowing (on Concept II ergometer)

50 watts, 16 mph								
age 20–29	4.0	4.4	4.9	5.4	5.9	6.4	6.8	7.3
age 30–39	3.6	4.0	4.4	4.8	5.3	5.7	6.1	6.5
age 40–49	3.4	3.8	4.2	4.6	5.0	5.4	5.8	6.2
110 watts, 16 mph								
age 20–29	7.3	8.2	9.0	9.4	9.9	10.2	10.9	11.7
age 30–39	7.3	8.2	9.0	9.9	10.8	11.6	12.5	13.4
age 40–49	6.8	7.7	8.5	9.3	10.8	11.6	12.5	13.4
Stationary ergometer								
General	8.3	9.3	10.3	11.3	12.3	13.3	14.3	15.3
Running								
6 mph, 10 min/hour pace	8.8	9.8	10.9	11.9	13.0	14.0	15.1	16.1
8.6 mph, 7 min/hour pace	12.3	13.7	15.2	16.7	18.1	19.6	21.1	22.5
In water, 1.3 m deep, no vest, maximum effort	15.0	16.8	18.6	20.4	22.2	24.0	25.8	27.5

Activity	Body weights (in lbs)							
	110	123	139	150	163	176	190	203
Jog-walk combo (jog portion less than 10 mins)	5.3	5.9	6.5	7.1	7.8	8.4	9.0	9.7
Skiing machines								
Nordic Trac (general)	8.3	9.3	10.3	11.3	12.3	13.3	14.3	15.3
Slide board								
66-in-wide board done to 40 slides/min	7.7	8.7	9.6	10.5	11.4	12.4	13.3	14.2
Stair climbing								
LifeStep 78% max heart rate	6.3	7.0	7.8	8.5	9.3	10.0	10.8	11.5
Stairmaster 4000								
30 steps/min	6.1	6.9	7.6	8.3	9.1	9.8	10.5	11.3
46–48 steps/min	8.8	9.8	10.9	11.9	13.0	14.0	15.1	16.1

Swimming							
Slow crawl, 50yds/min	7.0	7.8	8.7	9.5	10.4	11.2	12.0	12.9
Freestyle laps, vigorous effort	8.8	9.8	10.9	11.9	13.0	14.0	15.1	16.1
Tai chi							
Skilled performers	3.6	4.0	4.4	4.9	5.3	5.7	6.2	6.6
Tae kwan do	8.2	9.2	10.2	11.2	12.2	13.2	14.1	15.1
Tennis – recreational							
Doubles	6.1	6.9	7.6	8.3	9.1	9.8	10.5	11.3
Singles	7.0	7.8	8.7	9.5	10.4	11.2	12.0	12.9
Trampoline – recreational	3.1	3.4	3.8	4.2	4.5	4.9	5.3	5.6
Walking – general							
3 mph, level, firm surface	3.1	3.4	3.8	4.2	4.5	4.9	5.3	5.6
4 mph, level, firm surface	3.5	3.9	4.3	4.8	5.2	5.6	6.0	6.4
Wearing 1lb hand weight at 70% max heart rate	7.8	8.7	9.6	10.6	11.5	12.4	13.4	14.3

Activity	Body weights (in lbs)							
	110	123	139	150	163	176	190	203
Race walking								
6 mph	9.6	10.8	11.9	13.1	14.2	15.4	16.6	17.7
8 mph	14.0	15.7	17.4	19.0	20.7	22.4	24.1	25.8
Treadmill								
3 mph, no incline	4.0	4.5	4.9	5.4	5.9	6.4	6.9	7.3
4 mph, no incline	5.1	5.8	6.4	7.0	7.6	8.2	8.8	9.5
Yoga	3.0	3.3	3.7	4.0	4.4	4.8	5.1	5.5
Resistance training								
General circuit with machines	7.0	7.8	8.7	9.5	10.4	11.2	12.0	12.9
Universal gym	6.1	6.9	7.6	8.3	9.0	9.7	10.5	11.2
Nautilus – 12 exercises, 8–12 reps @ 14–19 min duration	4.1	4.6	5.1	5.6	6.1	6.6	7.1	7.6

Sports and fun

	3.9	4.4	4.9	5.4	5.8	6.3	6.8	7.2
Badminton	3.9	4.4	4.9	5.4	5.8	6.3	6.8	7.2
Baseball – non-game, shooting around	5.3	5.9	6.5	7.1	7.8	8.4	9.0	9.7
Bowling	2.6	2.9	3.3	3.6	3.9	4.2	4.5	4.8
Darts – wall or lawn	2.2	2.5	2.7	3.0	3.2	3.5	3.8	4.0
Frisbee	2.6	2.9	3.3	3.6	3.9	4.2	4.5	4.8
Golf – general	3.9	4.4	4.9	5.4	5.8	6.3	6.8	7.2
Golf – miniature	2.6	2.9	3.3	3.6	3.9	4.2	4.5	4.8
Juggling	3.5	3.9	4.3	4.8	5.2	5.6	6.0	6.4
Racquetball – casual	6.1	6.9	7.6	8.3	9.1	9.8	10.5	11.3
Soccer – casual	6.1	6.9	7.6	8.3	9.1	9.8	10.5	11.3
Softball – fast or slow pitch	4.4	4.9	5.4	6.0	6.5	7.0	7.5	8.1
Table tennis/ping-pong	3.5	3.9	4.3	4.8	5.2	5.6	6.0	6.4
Volleyball								
Beach	6.1	6.9	7.6	8.3	9.1	9.8	10.5	11.3
Indoors	2.6	2.9	3.3	3.6	3.9	4.4	4.7	5.0

Source: Calorie Expenditure Charts, by Frank Katch, Victor Katch and William McArdle, Fitness Technologies Press, 1996.

Calculating your exercise heart rate

If your age and corresponding exercise heart rate are not included in the chart on page 83 in Chapter Four, you can calculate the value yourself. Here's how:

1 Determine your maximum heart rate by subtracting your age from 220:

220 – _____ = _____
       your age   max heart rate

2 Multiply the number you get by the percentages below for heart rate zones:

Start-up rate = _____ × 0.55 = _____
           max heart rate   beats per minute

Intermediate = _____ × 0.65 = _____
           max heart rate   beats per minute

Experienced = _____ × 0.75 = _____
           max heart rate   beats per minute

Shape, tone and define those muscles

You took all those measurements of yourself back in Chapter Two, remember? Now it's time to adjust the numbers a bit. Losing lbs is only part of the solution to your figure flaws. Adding and subtracting inches are equally important.

Instead of aiming for the smallest waist possible or the tightest butt in the gym, you should instead focus on balancing your body proportions. Big hips don't look nearly as wide when matched by broad shoulders. That's why fashion designers put shoulder pads in jackets and dresses. Shapely, muscular calves draw the eye away from thick thighs. That's what high-heeled shoes have always done for women, in addition to killing our feet!

As discussed in Chapter Three, the 'X' in the H-O-A-X figure categories is based on the notion that to achieve the 'classic' hourglass figure, a woman's bust and hip measurements should be about the same, with a waistline that is 10 inches (25 cm) smaller. Take a look at your measurements and decide which ones have to be built up or scaled down to achieve these proportions. Then select some shaping, toning and defining exercises from the charts below to achieve those results.

Even if you're well proportioned or at your healthy body weight, flabby arms, jiggly thighs, or a pot-belly may still be a problem. You, too, must do some shaping, toning and defining exercises to control the loose flesh that will be revealed in an off-the-shoulder bridal gown or honeymoon bikini.

Then there are women who aren't really flabby – they just lack definition. You know who you are. Maybe your arms are tubular, your back is square and/or your calves straight. Well, that's all right if you're Mrs Potato Head, but ideally, real bodies have muscles with shapes and curves. You can use the shaping, toning and defining

THE TRUTH ABOUT CELLULITE

Some thin people have cellulite and some fat people don't – sort of like freckles. And as much as the money-hungry cosmetics industry would like you to believe you can rub a cream onto your thighs and make cellulite disappear, it's never going to happen, any more than you can wash away your freckles.

Cellulite is a dimpling of the skin caused by connective tissue stretching over fat cells. One of the ways to minimise the dimpling is to shrink the size of those fat cells so the connective tissue doesn't have to stretch so far. And isn't that just what you're trying to do anyway?

In addition to shrinking the fat cells, you also need to strengthen the muscles in the area of the dimpling, typically the hips, thighs and butt. Strong muscles are more rigid, which allows them to pull and smooth out the layer of fat, connective tissue and skin that lies on top of them.

exercises to chisel out some curves in your muscles just like a sculptor does in marble.

With the recommended exercises, you have the option of doing them at home with no special equipment, using inexpensive dumb-bells and barbells, or working out with free-standing resistance equipment. You can also take advantage of some common household items to help you with your workouts. Tins of soup (with the soup still inside, of course) can fill in for 1 lb hand weights or dumb-bells. A sturdy wooden box or the lower step of a staircase can serve as a bench. A chair back can replace the ballet barre and a 10-inch (25 cm) rubber ball can be used as a squeeze ball.

Exercises to shape, tone and define

The floor work exercises we refer to in the chart on page 124 are the ones you can do using your own body weight for resistance. For example, when you do a push-up, it's just you and your muscles down there on the floor. By using proper form and the right number of sets and repetitions, you can get results that are every bit as good as when expensive exercise equipment is used.

Most of these exercises can also be done using free weights, like dumb-bells and barbells or ankle and wrist weights. The common household items mentioned earlier can also be used as substitutes. By adding weights to your workout you can control the amount of resistance applied to a particular muscle and get better shaping and definition.

Resistance equipment is the stuff that you may find in your brother's bedroom or your fiancé's basement. A multipurpose bench, universal gym, fixed weight machines, or Nautilus and Cybex equipment fall into this category. Any gym or fitness centre you go to will be filled with the stuff.

Descriptions of the most basic exercises you can do without free weights or resistance equipment to shape, tone and define your muscles are provided after the chart. If you have your own 'heavy metal' or a gym membership, follow the instructions for form and technique provided with each piece you work out with.

Do it right or don't do it at all

One of the most common mistakes made when doing toning and resistance exercises is going too fast. The action, or work, should be very slow and deliberate so you can isolate the involved muscle and contract it through the entire motion, then slowly release it. There should be no bounce and swing in the movement, just a slow, concentrated contraction. If done properly, you won't be able to do as many repetitions, but you'll see results a lot sooner.

And remember, *exhale* on the exertion. Breathing during the exertion ensures that blood flow will not be blocked when you are working the muscle, which can lead to cramping. The abdominal muscles also contract when exhaling, which helps strengthen the abs in their flattened position.

As important as your speed is your form. Just because you're working on your biceps doesn't mean the rest of your muscles get to take a siesta. Before each exercise you must get into proper position. If standing, are your feet and legs shoulder-width apart with weight equally distributed? Are your shoulders squarely over your hips? Is your stomach pulled in? If you remember to check your alignment before each repetition, you'll get the benefit of toning all those other muscle groups while specifically working the one. See 'Pointers on Posture' later in this chapter for more tips to use during your workout.

Weight training should be done at least three days a week

and you should let muscles rest a day between training sessions. Four to five exercises should be done for both the upper and lower body muscles. Each set should include 10 to 15 repetitions, with 1 to 2 sets per workout.

How to do it

Many an injury has occurred in otherwise fit people who ignore the fundamental rules of exercise.

Do not take short cuts.

Use all exercise equipment properly or you risk being sidelined in these crucial weeks before the ceremony when you can least afford to be wrapped in bandages or hobbling on crutches.

Weight training exercises

	Floor work	Resistance equipment
Shoulders	Shrugs	Lateral raises
Upper back	Deltoid push-up	Back extension
Chest	Push-up	Butterfly machine
Triceps	Bench dip	Bench press
Biceps	Bicep curl	Lateral pulldown
Upper abs	Trunk curl	Ab press
Lower abs	Crunch	Ab press
Buttocks	Donkey kicks	Kneeling leg curl
Hips	Side squats	Hip machine
Thighs	Wall squat	Adduction/ abduction machines
Quadriceps	Lunges	Leg extension
Hamstring	Arabesque	Seated leg curl
Calves	Heel raise and toe ups	Leg presses
Waist	Side bends	Rotary torso

Abdominal crunch: lie on back with knees bent, feet flat on floor and hip-width apart, stomach muscles tight. Place hands behind your head, fingertips touching, but not linked. Keep elbows straight out to the sides of your head the entire time. Tuck chin slightly. Now slowly pull up your head, neck, shoulders and chest in one movement, pausing once your upper back is raised off the floor, then slowly lower yourself to the starting position. Repeat 8 to 12 times.

Arabesque: use a high-back chair for this exercise. Stand with feet hip-width apart and chair back in front of you an arm's length away. Slowly extend your left leg straight back, tightening the gluteal muscles as you raise your leg until it is 8 to 12 inches (20 to 30 cm) off the floor. Now slightly bend the knee to lift the heel towards your butt, while maintaining the contraction in the upper leg. Hold for 10 seconds, then extend the leg and slowly bring it back to the starting position. Repeat 8 to 12 times, then do the other leg.

TIP: Do a posture check – head up, shoulders and hips aligned, tummy pulled in.

Bench dips: find a bench or sturdy chair to use with this exercise. Sit on the edge of the bench with your legs together straight in front of you, toes pointing up. Grip the bench behind you with the heels of your hands. Keep your elbows relaxed, then slide your behind off the seat and support your weight with your arms. Slowly bend your elbows to lower your body until your upper arms are parallel to the floor behind you. Now slowly raise yourself back up again without settling back onto the seat. Repeat 8 to 12 times.

Bicep curls: use two 1 lb cans or dumb-bells for this exercise. Stand with feet shoulder-width apart, holding one weight in each hand with palms facing up. Pull the upper arms close to the body and pinch the elbows into your waist. Slowly raise your hands up to your shoulders, hold that position, then slowly lower your arms to your sides. Repeat 8 to 12 times.

Deltoid push-up: make your body into a bridge, bending at the waist, with your butt in the air, hands flat on the floor shoulder-width apart and legs together with your toes down and heels raised. Slowly lower your head to the floor by bending your elbows, hold the position, then slowly raise yourself back to the starting position. Repeat 8 to 12 times.

Donkey kick: get down on all fours on a padded carpet or exercise mat. Rest your weight on your forearms, with your palms down. Slowly pull your left knee into your chest, keeping your back straight – do not arch or hollow your back. Now slowly extend that leg out and above your buttocks pushing your heel towards the ceiling. Hold the position, then slowly bring the leg back under your body without putting your weight on it. Repeat 10 to 20 times, then do the other leg.

TIPS: Pull in your stomach to keep your back from sagging. Keep your head up and your neck aligned with your spine.

Forward lunges: stand with feet together, hands on hips. Extend left foot about two feet in front of you, planting foot firmly on floor, toes forward. Slowly lower your body to bring the right knee towards the floor. Keep your head up and your back straight. Stop when the knee of the front leg is at a right angle. Hold that position, then slowly raise your body up and bring in the front leg to the starting position. Repeat 8 to 12 times, then do the other leg.

TIPS: Squeeze your buttocks together and pull in your stomach with each lunge. Keep your head up and look straight in front of you, not at the floor.

Heel raises and toe ups: stand with feet together, hips and shoulders aligned. Hold onto a wall or chair back for balance. Raise your heels and curl onto your toes while tightening the buttocks and abdominal muscles. Hold for 3 to 5 seconds. Then lower to starting position. Repeat 10 to 20 times. Now flex your feet, raising your toes while you rock back onto your heels. Hold for 3 to 5 seconds. Return to start position. Repeat 10 to 20 times.

Tips: Tighten your buttocks and abdominal muscles as you raise and lower yourself. Don't look down. Keep your chest and head up.

Push-ups (beginners): lie on your stomach on a padded carpet or exercise mat. Place your hands underneath each shoulder, palms down. Bend your knees, about 8 to 10 inches (20 to 25 cm) apart, and cross your ankles in the air. Now slowly straighten your arms to lift your torso off the floor, keeping your weight balanced on your hands and knees. Pause once your body is raised, then slowly lower yourself until your upper arms are parallel to the floor – do not go all the way back to the starting position. Repeat 8 to 12 times.

TIPS: Keep back straight throughout the exercise. Tighten abs to support back and keep chin tucked.

Shoulder shrugs: use two 1 lb cans or dumbbells. Stand with feet hip-width apart, shoulders relaxed, arms down at your side, holding one weight in each hand. Slowly raise your shoulders straight up towards your ears, hold the position, then slowly lower them again. Repeat 10 to 20 times.

TIPS: Tuck buttocks beneath you and slightly tilt hips back. Exhale as you raise your shoulders, inhale when you lower them.

Side bends: use a 1 lb can or dumb-bell. Stand with feet shoulder-width apart, left arm at your side holding the weight. Put your right hand behind your head with your elbow sticking straight out from your ear. Bending at the waist, slowly slide your left hand towards the floor without tipping forward or shifting your pelvis. Your right elbow should point towards the ceiling as you dip to the left. Bend to the lowest point you can reach, hold, then slowly come up to the starting position. Repeat 10 to 20 times, then do the other side.

TIPS: Keep shoulders square and stomach pulled in. Proper form is more important than how far you can dip.

Side squats: stand with legs hip-width apart, feet facing forward, not turned out. Extend arms straight in front of you for balance, or rest them on your hips. Squat down about 8 to 12 inches (20 to 30 cm) by slowly bending the knees without tipping forward. Now step out to the left as far as you can, still holding the squat position. Pull the right leg over next to the left while in the squat, then slowly return to a standing position. Now repeat the movement, stepping out to the right first and bringing in your left leg. Repeat 10 to 12 times.

TIPS: Keep toes facing front at all times. Do not bounce down and up; control the movement from start to finish.

Trunk curl: lie on your back on a carpet or padded mat. Bend your knees and pull your feet in towards your butt. Now drop your knees out to the sides and put the soles of your feet together. Position your arms over the front of your body with your hands crossed over your waist. Slowly curl your shoulders and back off the floor without jerking your neck, and reach towards your ankles with your hands. Only your upper back should rise off the floor. Hold the position 10 seconds, then slowly lower your shoulders until your head is just above the floor. Repeat 8 to 12 times.

TIPS: Keep your head aligned with your spine and your chin up. Do not use your head and neck to pull yourself up.

Wall squats: stand about one foot away from wall with hands on hips. Lean back against the wall making sure head, shoulders and lower back are touching it. Slowly lower backside down the wall until you are in a sitting position with your knees at right angles. Hold the position, then slowly raise yourself up again without moving your feet or pulling away from the wall. Repeat 8 to 12 times.

TIPS: Keep weight evenly distributed on both legs to maintain balance. Don't lurch forward or remove head from contact with wall.

Working out with others

There is no one perfect time or place to work out. Different people have different tastes in this, just as they do with diamond settings. But if you are thinking about joining a gym, there are some things you should consider before signing on the dotted line.

How convenient is the gym to your home or job?

You're going to have to get there three or four times a week. It better be on the way to or from the place you travel to each day or you may never make it. Next, what are the hours of operation?

Beware of being oversold on the juice bar, tanning salon, childcare services and herbal shampoo if you have no intention of using them. If you're into classes like spinning, body pump or kickboxing, check out when they are scheduled, then visit when you're most likely to attend to see how crowded they are. If you're mainly interested in using the aerobic and resistance equipment, visit during the weekend hours you're likely to be using the gym and note how long the wait is to get on the pieces you want.

If you're thinking of hiring a personal trainer, the best way to find a good one is through direct referral from someone who has used a trainer and been satisfied with the results. It's just like finding a good photographer or band for your wedding. Once you have a name or two, be sure to verify that the person is a member of either the Association of Personal Trainers (0191 209 1031) or is on the National Register of Personal Trainers (0181 944 6688).

ONLINE TRAINING

Recently, we heard about an online personal trainer. At reasonable fees, personal trainer Paul Becker provides a diet plan, a training regimen and coaching online after you answer a series of questions about your eating habits, personal shape-up goals and more. Offline, Becker trains Los Angeles body builders, which we think is the reason he calls his company Truly Huge; in other words, that's not the lament of women who contact him for help with weight management and shaping up! For more info check out:

www.trulyhuge.com

One of the best ways to stick to a workout programme is to do it with an exercise buddy. Look at your *Wedding Dress Diet* 'Contract' to see if one of your 'supporters' is also someone who can work out with you. Once you've made a commitment to someone else to show up on the corner for that early-morning bike ride, or for regular Saturday-afternoon Rollerblading in the park, or for a lunchtime visit to the fitness centre in your office building, you'll be less likely to procrastinate about exercising. You have a date with someone and that's the commitment you keep, even if it's to go and exercise.

Resources and products we like

★ Exercise Association of England (08707 506 506)
★ Sports Council (0171 273 1500)
★ Sportsline (0171 222 8000)
★ Fitness Professionals (for information on 'Body Pump' weight training classes) (0990 133434)
★ Polar Heart Rate Monitor – several models and price ranges available (01926 816177) or www.polar.fi
★ Fitness Products – home exercise videos featuring aerobics, toning, stretching and much more (0171 704 2389)

Websites we like

★ www.active.org.uk British Health education authority website, designed to encourage people to 'get active for life'. Offers an analysis of your current activity level together with lots of suggestions for how to increase/improve this and how to have fun and variety while you're doing it.

★ www.get-motivated.com Get fit and get surfing with free Internet access from the first 'fitness portal' on the web. Get Motivated believe they have created the definitive website for anyone interested in health and fitness. Whether you want to find a personal trainer, gym, acupuncturist or masseur in your area, need new ideas for recipes or simply want to find out what's new and hot in the world of fitness – it's all here.

★ www.bodycontrol.co.uk Comprehensive site providing information on the Pilates method, how to find a teacher as well as purchase videos, books and clothing.

★ www. Boo.com is the first global Internet sports store. All merchandise is shown in 3D and can be viewed in minute detail down to the stitching! You can even try on your outfit on a mannequin your size in the virtual dressing room, complete with online sales assistant Miss Boo. Delivery is free and items should arrive within five days.

★ Two good exercise-related US websites are www.aceFitness.org and www.cooperaerobics.com.

Pointers on posture

Without counting a single calorie or lifting a single dumb-bell, you can lose 5 lbs. That is, the *illusion* of 5 lost lbs, but who's to know? The secret is good posture.

Ever catch your reflection in a store window or department store mirror and suddenly adjust yourself? If you answered 'yes', it's because you've seen how horrible the slumped shoulders and protruding belly look when you're slouching.

You can do something about that slouch and get rid of it forever. And there will never be a better time in your life than right now as you get ready to take centre stage on your wedding day. We're going to show you how.

Stand up with this book open in front of you and follow these simple instructions as you read them, then practise these steps every time you get up out of a chair or are standing for any length of time. You can condition your 'posture muscles' to remember what to do, just like all those soldiers have done before you. Don't think for a minute they all showed up at boot camp with straight spines and tight buns. If you follow this advice, you'll never have to make an adjustment in front of the mirror again!

★ Imagine yourself balancing a book on your head. If you do, you will straighten your back, raise your chest and ever so slightly lift the breasts.

★ Next, think about a swan or a graceful actress like Gwyneth Paltrow as you elongate your neck.

This keeps your chin up and prevents those dreadful doubles.

★ Now gently press your shoulders down and back to centre them over your hips. Be sure your weight is evenly distributed over each foot.

★ Finally, gently tighten the buttocks, which will also cause you to pull in those abdominal muscles.

Don't you feel lighter already?

Exercise myths and realities

. . . About **atrophy:** this is the shrinking of a muscle due to lack of use. The point is, muscle cannot turn into fat. Lack of exercise reduces the size of your muscles while increasing the opportunity for fat storage.

. . . About **breathing:** pay attention to your breathing when doing resistance exercises. Holding your breath when contracting a muscle causes you to push out the stomach muscles, which is where they're going to stay if you do it over and over. Exhale on the exertion and your stomach will compress.

. . . About **cooling down:** this is what you do at the end of an aerobic or a fast-paced resistance workout that raises heart rate. You're going to need that heart for the rest of your life. Give it a chance to return to a normal rhythm.

. . . About **dancing:** ballroom, jitterbug, salsa – it's all aerobic and a fun way to work out with your future husband. Sign up for some dance lessons so you can strut your stuff at the wedding. And don't forget to do some discreet stretches before you get on that dance floor at the wedding or you'll be hobbling on your honeymoon!

. . . About **fingers:** they can get smaller when you lose weight, which will affect your ring size. Don't take a chance on losing your wedding band while waving goodbye to your family at the airport. Have your rings refitted and, if necessary, resized a few weeks before the big day.

. . . About **gear:** we're not talking fashion here, but practical, comfortable clothing and sneakers. Don't forget your wristwatch with a second-hand sweep, heart monitor, hair clips, weight gloves and headset or portable music system.

. . . About **plateaux:** they happen, and they can be frustrating. The key to preventing them and breaking them is change. Vary your workouts by cross-training or doing circuit training. Break up long workouts by doing 3 different aerobic exercises for 15 minutes each instead of just one for 45 minutes. If you normally work out indoors, go outside and do something, or vice versa.

. . . About **reps:** as in repetitions, or how many times you repeat a particular exercise. Depending on your goal, you may increase your reps using a lighter resistance to tone a muscle, or limit the reps while using more resistance to increase the size of a muscle. The ideal number is one more than you can comfortably do with the given resistance. For example, when using a 3 lb dumb-bell to do bicep curls, if you can complete 9 in proper form and the 10th one takes maximum effort, stop at 10. Do more sets of these to tone, or increase the resistance and do fewer reps and sets to build muscles.

. . . About **sets:** how many times you repeat a series of exercises. For example, if you are working your upper body and doing 6 different exercises for 8 to 12 reps each, doing 2 or 3 more sets will provide better definition of the targeted muscles.

. . . About **stretching:** watch a cat and you'll understand what this is all about: slow, easy movements that give the muscles a chance to elongate and arch and relax. Best part of any workout!

. . . About **warming up:** do this before you start any type of workout. It's a necessary part of the whole exercise routine and you're a fool if you skip it. Start moving all the large muscle groups in a rhythmic pattern, slowly at first, then gradually progressing in speed. Marching in place while pumping the arms or side steps while swinging the arms out to each side will get the heart pumping and the blood flowing to those muscles you're about to work.

. . . About **water:** drink before you work out, while you work out and after you're finished working out. Aim for one litre of water per hour of exercise.

Exercising while doing other things

If you want to lose lbs and inches as quickly as possible, the exercising you need to do is what we've prescribed so far. However, we realise that not all brides-to-be can fit in the time for serious exercise – if they have, say, a couple of kids to care for, or they're forced to work 12-hour days at the office. If you're in a similar situation, you should incorporate what researchers call 'lifestyle' exercise into your daily routine. Lifestyle exercise includes activities such as walking around the house during the adverts on TV, or getting off the bus one stop earlier. Researchers at the Cooper Institute of Aerobics Research in Dallas recently concluded a study in which half of the participants spent 20 to 60 minutes per day up to 5 days a week vigorously exercising (swimming or

---

HOUSEWORK BURNS

If you perform household tasks vigorously, you are getting beneficial exercise. Window washing, food shopping, or mopping the floor burns 3.7 calories per minute. Sweeping or dusting uses 3.8 calories per minute. Waxing or scrubbing floors is good for 6.8 calories a minute. Vacuuming is a real workout: 7 calories per minute. Rake leaves – you'll burn 5 calories a minute.
  Remember, the key word here is *vigorously*.

bicycling, for example). The other half incorporated 30 minutes a day of lifestyle exercising. At the end of 6 months, researchers found that both groups had similar and significant improvements in cholesterol readings, blood pressure and body fat percentages. But – and this is key – *the lifestyle exercisers had to exercise three times longer than those who vigorously exercised in order to burn the same number of calories.* But we're talking about the wimpy lifestyle stuff here, like walking around during the adverts. The more vigorous tasks you perform regularly really can add points in your weekly calorie-burning goal. See 'Housework Burns' box.

Toners

And here are some toners you can do while doing something else, as well:

For tightening the abdominal muscles to flatten your stomach: Jacqueline got this tip from fitness expert Sheila Cluff: Just 'hold it in'. 'Make a habit of contracting your abdominal muscles whenever you think about it,' Cluff said. 'You can do this exercise any place and at any time – while cooking dinner, for example.' Contract your stomach muscles for a slow count of ten, relax and repeat, remembering to check and correct your posture at the same time and to breathe deeply.

To tone up the butt: another tip from Sheila Cluff: whenever you climb the stairs, pretend you're holding a gold coin between your cheeks and don't 'drop' it till you reach the top. A woman we know – who doesn't have stairs at home – does a lesser but still effective variation of this. Whenever she's doing 'hold it in' for her stomach, she also clenches her buttocks. She says she does this constantly when she's standing in a queue. 'As long as you're wearing a fairly full dress, a long loose-fitting skirt, or a big T-shirt over leggings, no one's the wiser!'

To trim the thighs: do wall squats – described earlier in this chapter – while you're on the phone. And here's another one of Sheila Cluff's funny but effective ideas, as long as you have stairs: waddle up the stairs with a wiggle like Charlie Chaplin, feet turned outwards, your knees flexed, your pelvis tucked. This is excellent for the inner thighs.

> *And don't forget the most fun exercise-while-doing-something-else activity of all: sex!*

See Chapter Ten for the calorie-burning potential!

CHAPTER SIX

Eating Between Fittings

By this time, you're probably feeling overwhelmed by all that you still have to do, and under-appreciated for all you have done so far. Eating right and exercising regularly may feel like more hassles in your already harried life. But you cannot give up!

*L*ook at it this way: You have to eat, right? If you give in to temptation at every turn, you will have to deal with all the guilt and lbs that follow. If you keep your wits about you, you can go to bed at night knowing you are a few ounces closer to your wedding-day weight. That's sure to lead to pleasant dreams!

Meals versus snacks

The worst mistake you can make is to skip a meal to make time for one more errand. No one ever lost weight by skipping meals. In fact, most people gain weight from all the meals they don't eat. Why? Because something will eventually cross your lips in lieu of the missed bowl of cereal or bowl of soup or plate of salad. And that something will, more likely than not, be something with more calories, fat and sodium than the meal you passed up.

The problem stems from the arbitrary way people categorise food. We think that if it's a 'mealtime', we eat 'meal food'. And if it's 'snack time' we eat 'snack food'.

Robyn has counselled many people who say they never have time for breakfast, yet they eat a stack of biscuits at around 3 pm 'for a snack'. It never occurs to them to have two pieces of toast and marmite at three o'clock, or a dish of porridge with raisins, both of which are lower in fat and calories than the biscuits. People are amazed to learn that the 'meal' they missed first thing in the morning can still be eaten in the middle of the afternoon. It's not as if your stomach can tell what time it is, or that the Food Police will arrest you for eating 'breakfast food' in the afternoon!

Another danger in skipping meals is that it is harder to keep track of all the 'little' things you eat as snacks. Meals are eaten at a table or another traditional 'eating place'. You set out dishes and plates in a ceremonial fashion, then place all the food in front of you. If you are eating with others, you're probably not doing anything else except talking while you eat. When you're finished, you have a pretty good idea of what you ate because you were paying attention to the food.

On the other hand, when you don't eat meals and snack your way through the day instead, you lose sight of what you have eaten within seconds after swallowing. Try going through your waste basket at the end of a day in which you skipped lunch. Count the food wrappers you find in there. Or look around your car after spending the day running to every shoe store and lingerie shop in town. There's bound to be evidence of food eaten that you have long since forgotten.

The bottom line is that

foods gobbled up while talking on the phone, driving the car and dashing through shopping precincts are lethal.

Such food is typically high in calories, fat and sodium, and it's too easy to forget to add it to your food log. Trust us, you're better off eating meals.

Okay, so you're going to eat a meal away from home. Well the bad news is you have to be careful here as well. In a recent study, researchers at the University of Memphis and Vanderbilt University found that women who eat more than five meals a week outside the home consume more calories, sodium and fat than those who eat out less often. The researchers found that women who ate out more often consumed an average of 2,056 calories a day, 3,299 mgs of sodium a day and obtained nearly 35 per cent of their daily calories from fat. The comparable data for the women who ate out less often: 1,768 calories, 2,902 mgs of sodium and 31 per cent of calories from fat. When asked about the implications of this data, the researchers rather wimpily replied that 'further research is needed to enhance healthful eating in restaurants'. Well, you don't have time to wait for that!

Keeping score

If your schedule looks crazy and you fear you might end up eating meals on the move, here's what to do:

1. Consider what your dining options are wherever you're going to be at a mealtime. Will you be in a department store, shopping precinct, on the motor-

way, or dropping something off at a friend's house? What kind of food is available to you that might meet your needs?

2. Subtotal your food log for the day so far *before* you leave home, work, or wherever you've spent the first part of your day. How many calories do you have left to work with? How many servings of fruits and vegetables, wholegrains and calcium-rich dairy foods have you eaten so far?

3. Decide ahead of time where you will eat your next meal. Change your route or the order in which you do your errands to make it possible to be near an eatery that has suitable choices.

4. Plan your menu so you know exactly what you will order when you get there. Use the guidelines below to help make your decision.

5. Record the meal on your food log as soon as you finish eating, then go about your business.

When eating commercially prepared food, you not only have to watch out for jumbo portions that will push up your calorie count, but also many hidden sources of fat and way too much sodium. That excess sodium won't put any permanent lbs on you, but you may feel puffy and swollen for a few days afterwards, which won't do much for your morale if you happen to have a fitting.

The recommendations that follow will help you make the most of your meals on the run.

Breakfast

Beware of the seemingly benign but secretly villainous breakfast sandwich

– that is, eggs and cheese plus ham, bacon, or sausage in a baguette or croissant. These sandwiches range from 400 to 800 calories and contain half a day's fat allowance. It's hard to believe that something as light and fluffy as a croissant can be fattening but it can carry up to 25 more grams of fat than an English muffin. Opt instead for an English muffin or toast and an order of scrambled eggs. Another alternative is a single box of cereal with low-fat milk.

Another seemingly innocent breakfast item is a bagel. The average bagel has 320 calories before you add the cream cheese or butter, which adds another 100 to 200 calories of pure fat. Right behind the bagel is the muffin. The typical raisin bran, or apple-cinnamon variety from the coffee bar can pack up to 500 calories with 25 grams of fat. You're better off getting a fruit smoothie and two slices of raisin bread topped with jam. Or go for a low-fat muesli bar, a container of yogurt and a banana for 300 calories and 3 grams of fat.

Food court in the shopping precinct

Approach this area just like you would a buffet (see the tips on this in Chapter Seven). You've got to see what your choices are and avoid the hype of 'combo specials' and 'super-sized meal deals'. You may get your best calorie-conscious deal by buying part of your meal at one counter and the rest at another.

The biggest source of calories in the food court is usually the meat, whether it's a hamburger, hot dog, or piece of fried chicken. You're better off skipping the meat and finding a vegetable meal you can enjoy; get your protein at another time and place where you can have better quality control.

A large baked potato will have about 300 calories, no fat and only 25 mg of sodium but watch out for those fatty toppings like cheese and bacon bits. Your best bets for toppings are baked beans or cottage cheese.

At the Chinese food counter, one cup of broccoli and bean curd with a cup of plain white rice will provide about 350 calories with 5 grams of fat and 100 mg of sodium if you don't add any additional soy sauce. Chicken chow mein is also a reasonable choice at 255 calories and 10 grams of fat per cup, but the sodium can go over 500 mg.

If there is a salad bar, it is worth checking out. What you want is lots of garden-variety vegetables with plain tuna or chicken on top and a low-fat or non-fat salad dressing. Skip the pasta, cheeses and olives.

Another great option is a couple of sushi rolls at about 150 calories each, no fat and less than 100 mg of sodium. Be cautious about dipping sauces, however.

Tips for other concessions in the food court and for all those freestanding fast-food places in other locations follow.

Fast-food burgers

Your best bet here is the kiddie burger with its small dollops of ketchup and mustard. Cheese can add another 100 calories and 8 grams of fat, so try to avoid it. Find some kind of side salad to go with your burger instead of the fries. Even a small fat-free frozen yogurt is a wiser choice than the fries.

Forget the deluxe burgers with 'double anything' and special sauces or extra toppings like bacon and cheese. These are not good foods for brides or for anyone else who is going to be trying on a custom-fitted dress in the near future.

Chicken

The key words here are roasted or 'grilled', *not* 'fried'. Beyond that, avoid the skin, pay extra for white meat if you must and ask for your chicken sandwich without sauce or mayonnaise.

Pizza

The pizza shop has more potential than most people realise. A single slice of cheese pizza with a thin crust has about 275 calories and 5 grams of fat. It's the second or third slice that can get you into trouble. Ask for a side order of vegetable toppings or a cup of minestrone soup to keep you from reaching for those additional slices. And, of course, steer clear of meat toppings, double crust, cheese-in-the-crust and deep-dish features.

Sandwiches

Some of the chains and supermarkets are making it easier to order sensibly because they've added lower-calorie and lower-fat sandwiches. If no such specially labelled menu items are available, go for the turkey breast; next best, roast beef; third best, boiled ham. If you can pass up the cheese, you'll save 100 calories per slice. Same goes for the mayonnaise, at 100 calories per tablespoon. Ask for whole wheat or wholegrain bread, and feel free to pile on the shredded lettuce, sliced tomato, onions, roasted peppers and any other vegetables on hand.

Proceed with caution at the sight of tortilla 'wraps' and 'stuffed' pittas. Most contain more high-fat dressing and cheese than you might realise, and those wraps and pittas are much higher in calories than two slices of bread.

Popular restaurant chains

Once you're looking at a printed menu instead of a lighted menu board, your choices will undoubtedly be better. Scan every section for foods you can put together to make a meal. A combination of appetisers and side dishes may do the job instead of an entrée. It is also a good idea to look for any healthy heart symbols among the menu choices.

An important way you'll save calories is to order *à la carte*. As economical as the early-bird special and complete meal prices might seem, they will probably cost you more calories than you can afford at present. Decide what you want and order only that.

> **Many a dish of ice cream has been eaten simply because it was included with the dinner!**

Don't expect too much help in the way of substitutions or special preparation in these chain restaurants. The menus are almost always inflexible, save say, allowing you to substitute sliced tomatoes for the french fries. Count on having to ask a lot of questions about how things are served and on scraping off the sauces and coatings you don't want to eat.

Delicatessen/deli counter

A real advantage here is that you pay for most items by weight. You can actually order 3 ounces of turkey breast and a $1/4$ of a pound of coleslaw and get just that. You can also buy a single banana and an 8-ounce carton of cottage cheese.

The prepared hot foods in these places are generally not diet-friendly. But the rotisserie chicken is (you can remove the skin for further calorie and fat savings), along with the fresh vegetables and fruit salads. Single-serving portions of condiments like low-fat mayonnaise and salad dressing are helpful, too.

You can have a sandwich made to order on the wholegrain bread or roll of your choice and have it piled high with roasted peppers, sliced mushrooms and bean sprouts if the spirit moves you. It's all there for the asking.

Stroll down the aisles for a box of low-fat muesli bars or a box of unsalted rice cakes to munch on later in the day, if needed. Then pick up a pack of gum or a roll of mints in the checkout line to pop in your mouth after one muesli bar so that you won't eat the whole box!

Convenience stores

These can be a challenge if you never go past the most convenient, ready-to-eat items on display at the front of the store. You do have other options. Just past the hamburgers and doughnuts you'll find a freezer case. Look for a healthy-style frozen entrée and pop it in the store's microwave for a quick lunch.

Get past the shelves stocked with crisps and dips and you'll find other shelves stocked with canned goods you can use, like tuna in brine, apple sauce and baked beans. There are also boxes of cereal, raisins and water biscuits – all low in fat. Then stroll by the refrigerated cases for yogurt and cottage cheese.

Right around the corner from the chocolate you'll find popcorn and fruit-filled cereal bars. Just keep your eyes open and don't be impulsive. Since nearly every food in the store has a label on it, read the nutrition facts before making any decision and you'll be fine.

Salad bars

A salad bar may seem like a no-brainer place to get a safe meal, but there are some fat traps even here. Walk past anything covered in mayonnaise, like potato or macaroni salad and tuna, ham, or egg salad. You also don't want to linger too long in front of the crispy Chinese noodles, seasoned croutons and sunflower seeds.

Focus on all things from Mother Nature's garden: mixed greens, shredded carrots and cabbage, sliced cucumbers and radishes, pepper strips or rings, raw onion rings and broccoli florets. Garnish with a light sprinkling of grated cheese, or cubed ham, or prawns.

Then, to top it all off, take advantage of the low-calorie dressing or your own vinaigrette with lots of balsamic vinegar and a splash of olive oil.

Okay, now you know what to eat when you're out and about on your own. But, as your wedding grows ever closer, what do you do when well-meaning friends, relatives and colleagues lure you to calorie-laden celebrations in your honour? You don't want to be rude. You don't want to be ungrateful. You don't want to spoil anyone's fun.

But you don't want a bigger butt, either!
Read on!

CHAPTER SEVEN

Showered with Calories

As if you didn't have enough 'on your plate' right now: getting the right addresses on the invitations, choosing presents for your bridesmaids, deciding on the food for your reception and trying to lose weight, your family and friends will heap on more.

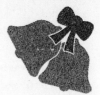

J In the final month before your wedding, you'll be fêted at successive parties with colleagues, girlfriends, bridesmaids and extended family where you must be the gracious guest of honour. The date, time and place of each event will often be out of your control, and the menu pre-set. And then of course there's your hen night! These situations can spell diet disaster if you don't have a game plan at the ready to bail you out. Here's what you need to know.

Rule 1: It is easier to control your surroundings than to control your behaviour.

★ When possible, position yourself as far from the food as you can. If you are sitting in front of a table laden with crips and dips, salted nuts, or chocolate dipped strawberries you can't be expected to ignore them. If they are across the room, you won't be as likely to eat them.

★ Suggest a restaurant that you know has a 'safe' menu. It's impossible to eat sensibly when your only choice is a burger and fries.

★ Stay out of the kitchen and canteen and away from vending machines and other food traps when stressed out, overtired, or otherwise out of sorts.

You will use food to medicate your emotions if it's nearby, so don't go near it.

Rule 2: Know what you are eating before you put anything in your mouth.

★ Look up serving size and caloric information first and then decide if you can afford to eat the food. It is too late to substitute a ham and salad on granary for the cheese and tuna melt once you've taken the last bite.

★ Ask questions about menu items and make your preferences clear before placing your order. Marinated vegetables can be swimming in olive oil or in balsamic vinegar. The difference is crucial to your calorie count.

Rule 3: Record everything you eat immediately after you eat it.

★ With so much going on in your life, don't expect your short-term memory to be as sharp as it was in your carefree, pre-engagement days. The side dish of coleslaw or croutons accompanying your salad can add another 100 calories to a meal. Keep a small notepad in your purse or grab a cocktail napkin off the table and jot down exactly what and how much you ate before leaving the restaurant or party.

Use these additional suggestions when attending specific functions in your honour.

Lunch with colleagues

★   Call home and cancel any dinner plans you might have had. You don't need two big meals in one day. Have a salad or bowl of vegetable soup that night.

★   If given a choice of where to go for the lunch, suggest a diet-friendly place, like a Thai, Japanese, or Middle Eastern restaurant.

★   Opt for a fruit juice spritzer instead of an alcoholic beverage to help keep your wits about you when the ordering begins.

★   Check the appetiser menu for possible lunch options, like a seafood cocktail and grilled vegetables.

★   Pose for a picture with each of your friends around the table so you're less likely to nibble on the shared chicken wings and crispy potato skins and sour cream.

★   If you receive cards and gifts, start to open them when the food is served and be sure to read each card out loud. You'll be too busy to do much eating.

★   Definitely share dessert, then don't eat your share.

In all of the charts that follow, we provide the average calorie value of each food item since there may be many versions of the food. The serving sizes are typical, but your actual portion size may vary.

Lunch with colleagues

Diet disasters

	Calories	Serving
Regular beer	150	12 fl oz (350 ml)
Rum & Coke	200	8 fl oz (250 ml)
Wine spritzer	100	12 fl oz (350 ml)
Nacho platter	350	6–8 pieces
Spicy chicken wings	450	4 pieces
Potato skins	300	4 pieces
Cream of tomato soup	160	8 fl oz (250 ml)
Vegetable beef soup	175	8 fl oz (250 ml)
Tuna salad sandwich	500	average
Hamburger on bun	500	average
Chef salad with Russian dressing	600	
Carrot cake with cream cheese frosting	475	
Chocolate brownie	250	per 2 × 2 × 1-inch (5 × 5 × 2.5 cm) piece

Diet dreams

	Calories	Serving
Light beer	100	12 fl oz (350 ml)
Diet Coke	1	12 fl oz (350 ml)
Seltzer with lime	0	
California roll	120	6-inch (15 cm) roll
Hummus & pitta triangles	150	50g hummus plus 4 triangles
Steamed artichoke	60 each	
Gazpacho	60	8 fl oz (250 ml)
Minestrone	85	8 fl oz (250 ml)
Bacon, lettuce & tomato	350	average
Garden burger on bun	275	average
Spinach salad with vinaigrette	350	
Madeira cake	200	per 1-inch (2.5 cm) slice
Chocolate biscotti	100	1 oz (25 g) or 5 × 1-inch (12 × 2.5 cm) piece

Hen night

Diet disasters

	Calories	Serving
Black Russian	275	8 fl oz (250 ml)
Gin & tonic	175	8 fl oz (250 ml)
Pina colada	370	8 fl oz (250 ml)
Guacamole & crisps	250	2 oz (50 g) dip and 1 oz (25 g) crisps
Fried aubergine	250	10 oz (250 g)
Egg roll	180	each
Beef & bean enchilada	400	each
Chicken lo mein	400	8 oz (225 g)
Refried beans	250	10 oz (250 g)
Fried mozzarella sticks and tomato	450	5 pieces
Fried rice	375	5 oz (125 g)
Ice cream	400	8 fl oz (180 g)
Cheesecake	450	slice
Almond cookie	45	each

Diet dreams

	Calories	Serving
Fat-free latte	40	8 fl oz (250 ml)
Scotch & soda	100	8 fl oz (250 ml)
Screwdriver	175	8 fl oz (250 ml)
Salsa & chips	160	2 oz (50 g) dip and 1 oz (25 g) crisps
Roasted vegetables	100	8 oz (225 g)
Wonton soup	80	8 fl oz (250 ml)
Beef fajitas	250	each
Chicken chow mein	250	8 oz (225 g)
Black bean soup	125	8 fl oz (250 ml)
Sliced mozzarella, ½ tomato plus vinaigrette	200	2 oz (50 g)
White rice	160	5 oz (125 g)
Sorbet	200	8 fl oz (190 g)
Zabaglione	160	serving
Fortune cookie	25	each

Hen night

❤ Spend that afternoon in your bikini or sexiest and smallest piece of lingerie to fortify your will-power not to indulge.

❤ Wear something clingy, fitted, or belted for a constant reminder not to overeat.

❤ Order a fat-free latte, it'll look like you're drinking a Black Russian, but with far fewer calories.

❤ Avoid bar snacks. They're usually smothered in salt, make you thirsty and you'll end up drinking even more.

❤ If you do end up toasting your own health along with the girls, order a non-alcoholic drink in between each full proof one to dilute the damage.

❤ When it's time to order, suggest you share appetisers around the table, then simply skip your turn after one or two samples when the plates come your way.

❤ Do not ask for a doggy bag unless you really have a dog and really plan on giving the rest of that pasta to him or her. You don't need it.

The surprise hen party

❤ Slip into the kitchen and pour yourself a big glass of water after the initial glare of flashbulbs and tears of surprise have passed. Drink the entire thing to help fill yourself up before you re-enter the party.

- ❤ Mingle, socialise and greet all your long-lost friends. It will keep you talking rather than eating.

- ❤ Put some munchies on a party napkin or small plate and limit yourself to eating only those. Don't eat any hors d'oeuvres directly from the serving tray and platters – it's too hard to keep track of how much you've had.

- ❤ This is a good time to opt for a 'virgin' drink like plain tomato juice or orange juice with a twist.

- ❤ Don't let your well-meaning hostess 'fix a plate' for you. Get in line with everyone else and make your own selections.

- ❤ Practise saying 'thank you' when given a present and 'no thank you' when offered another dessert.

- ❤ Decline the offer to take home the other half of the cake or the remains of your friend Claire's Coronation chicken. Tell them your refrigerator is broken and you have nowhere to store it.

Menu items	Calories	Serving
Party punch	200	8 fl oz (250 ml)
Mixed nuts	200	3 oz (75 g)
Spinach dip and bread	100	2 oz (50 g), 4 bread cubes
Finger sandwiches	100	each
Devilled eggs	75	half egg
Tossed salad with Italian dressing	50	1 oz (25 g)
Petits fours	85	each

Tasting night at the caterer's

❤ Scrutinise the full menu in advance and circle those items that you must make a decision about so as to avoid eating things you weren't planning to serve anyway.

❤ Sample each item as if you were a food critic – get the essence of the taste and texture in the first bite.

❤ Take as many people along as you are permitted and let them cast their votes on the food so you don't have to try everything.

❤ Be the stenographer, keeping track of what was served and what the comments were. You'll be too busy to overeat.

❤ Don't sample anything that is not dependent on the chef's culinary skills, such as the salad, assorted cheeses and crackers, raw shellfish, baked potatoes, melon balls, etc.

❤ Dip the tines of a fork into any dressings or dips you wish to taste.

❤ Step into the ladies' room midway through the evening and run cold water over your wrists to revive your numbed senses after an hour of sampling.

The rehearsal dinner

❤ Try on your honeymoon outfit that afternoon as a reminder of how great you look after all your hard work.

- ❤ Be sure to eat before going to the rehearsal since it often takes longer than anyone planned and you don't want to arrive at the restaurant starving.
- ❤ Limit yourself to one alcoholic drink to toast the occasion – preferably with your meal, not before.
- ❤ Order something you like, but not a favourite dish. You'll be less inclined to gobble up every bite.
- ❤ Be sure to sit next to your fiancé and pass off any unwanted food onto his plate.
- ❤ When prodded to order an appetiser or to eat more food than you want to, refuse by confessing that you are really nervous and feel like bumble bees are buzzing around inside your stomach.

Menu items	Calories	Serving
Red or white wine	100	4 fl oz (120 ml)
French onion soup	30	8 fl oz (250 ml)
with melted cheese and bread	+150	
French bread	50	2 oz (50 g) slice
with butter	+35	teaspoon
Mesclun salad	10	1 oz (25 g)
with French dressing	+50	tablespoon
Broiled flounder	200	6 oz (150 g)
Boiled new potatoes	100	3 potatoes
roasted in olive oil	+100	
Asparagus	25	6 spears
with hollandaise sauce	+50	2 tablespoons
Crème brûlée	>200	5 oz (125 g)

- To shave calories, avoid 'add ons' in the form of sauces, spreads, dressings, stuffings and toppings.
- Watch out for high-salt items like soups, tomato sauce, barbecue sauce, ham and anything with soy sauce on it. You can't afford to be bloated this close to the wedding.

How to navigate a buffet

- Walk up, down and around all of the serving tables, including the dessert stand, to see what is being served. Then predetermine exactly what you're going to eat from the available choices.
- If something looks fabulous but fattening, go ahead and have a small portion, but don't waste any calories on foods you can get any time, such as potato salad or chicken wings.
- If there isn't an 'undressed' salad, make one for yourself out of the garnishes. Look for things like pepper rings, cherry tomatoes, kale, radish roses, parsley and orange slices.
- Eat in courses, just as if you were dining *à la carte*, and sit down to eat each course before returning to the line for more. With any luck, the line will be too long to bother getting up again, or the food will run out and you won't be able to eat as much.
- Use a salad or dessert plate for your selections and you'll have to take smaller portions.

❤ Choose a table as far from the buffet as possible to make the trip back more difficult.

❤ Don't let anyone else bring you any food while he or she is at the buffet.

❤ Do not eat anything off your plate while moving through the line, not even a stray cheese cube.

❤ Visit the ladies' room after your plate is cleared and brush your teeth or rinse your mouth with mouthwash to diminish the desire for dessert. Almost everything tastes awful when you have a minty mouth.

❤ Never weigh yourself the day after a meal like this – it will only weaken your resolve. Most buffet and banquet foods are covered with salty sauces to keep them from drying out. You will undoubtedly retain fluid for a few days after eating them, which will show up on your scales as water weight – but it will pass.

The wedding day

❤ Eat slowly and signal the waiter to clear your plate before you've finished.

❤ Stay hydrated with water – it's a long day of dancing and posing and lugging around that gown.

Menu items	Calories	Serving
Champagne	80	4 fl oz (120 ml)

APPETISERS

Menu items	Calories	Serving
Stuffed mushroom	50	each
Mini quiche	75	each
Cheese puff	100	each
Spinach wrapped in filo pastry	125	each

FIRST COURSES

Menu items	Calories	Serving
Caesar salad	100	1 oz (25 g)
Fresh fruit cocktail with sorbet	150	serving
Cream of mushroom soup	160	8 fl oz (250 ml)

MAIN COURSE ENTREES

Menu items	Calories	Serving
Lobster tail	150	6 oz (150 g)
Grilled salmon	300	6 oz (150 g)
Chicken cordon bleu	450	serving
Prime rib	800	8 oz (200 g)

SIDE STARCHES

Menu items	Calories	Serving
Wild rice pilaf	120	3 oz (75 g)
Cloverleaf roll with butter	150	each
Bread stuffing	180	3 oz (75 g)
Twice-baked stuffed potato	275	serving

Glazed carrots	50	5 oz (125 g)
Green beans with almonds and butter sauce	80	5 oz (125 g)
Peas with mushrooms and cream sauce	100	4 oz (100 g)

DESSERTS

Coffee with cream and sugar	30	8 fl oz (250 ml)
Chocolate-covered strawberry	60	each
Two-layer cake with buttercream	300	1 in (2.5 cm) slice

LIQUEURS

Crème de menthe	185	1½ oz (30–49 ml)

Post-reception room service in the bridal suite

❤ Tantalise one another with blissfully low-calorie foods of love, such as peeled, seedless grapes, oysters, fresh raspberries and caviar on toast triangles.

❤ Put on your sexiest, skimpiest negligee and eating won't even cross your mind!

Menu items	Calories	Serving
Raw oysters	50	med.
Caviar	40	tablespoon
Toast points	20	each triangle
Seedless grapes	80	20 individual grapes
Raspberries	60	5 oz (125 g)
Camembert cheese	85	1 oz (25 g)
Brie	95	1 oz (25 g)
Water biscuits	30	2 pieces

CHAPTER EIGHT

Setting Up a Slim Kitchen

Is your kitchen co-operating? Is it adapting to your new healthy eating habits? If not, put it on a diet. Don't let it tempt you with that half bag of chocolate buttons you ostensibly keep for baking.

*D*on't let it beckon you to the freezer for that cheese-laden lasagne. Throw that stuff out. Do a kitchen 'remodel' – not just to make your life easier while you're dieting, but to help you maintain your weight loss and your healthy eating style once you weigh what you want to. Let us count the simple and (mostly) inexpensive ways.

Slim-conscious cookware and gadgets

If you can't afford these items right now, why not put some of them on your wedding list?

Bamboo steamers: use them on top of a pot of boiling water to steam vegetables and other foods; cooking oil isn't necessary. Steaming retains nutrients that are often lost during conventional cooking. The steamers come in various sizes to accommodate different pots, and they're interesting-looking enough that you can hang them on the wall, if they fit in with your kitchen decor or if storage space is a problem.

Crock pot or pressure cooker: both allow you to cook meat and/or vegetables without losing nutrients and in liquid instead of oil.

Extra ice cube trays: use them to freeze stock, egg whites, fruit purees, sauces, etc.

Fat separator: usually in the form of a measuring cup, this nifty gadget makes the fat from the juices of meat or poultry float to the top. Open a valve on the bottom to release the fat-free juices, then use the juices to moisturise and flavour the cooked meat. Many models will also allow you to separate egg whites from yolks, a requirement in many low-fat recipes.

Food processors: these will save you a lot of time as you add more fruits and veggies to your diet. Larger models are great for chopping and slicing. Mini processors are just right for tackling small but time-consuming tasks like chopping herbs and garlic and grating cheese.

Garlic press: another way to make the most of this pungent, tasty, healthy bulb. The best models have a stainless-steel press screen that pivots out for easy cleaning and a comfortable, ergonomic plastic handle.

Kitchen sprouter: all you need are some seeds, a little water and a few days to grow sprouts in your kitchen for your salads and vegetable dishes.

Non-stick pans and baking trays: going non-stick is one of the most dramatic ways to cut your fat intake. Consider that when you cook with a conventional pan, you must use several tablespoons of oil or other fat, while with a non-stick pan a teaspoon – or a single squirt of a non-stick cooking spray – will suffice. The average tablespoon of cooking oil (and remember, you may need several) has about 14 grams of fat and 122 calories. When you cut back to a teaspoon, each of those numbers is reduced by two-thirds. A general rule when buying non-stick cookware: opt for the heaviest you can afford.

Oil sprayer: fill this device with olive oil or another oil and it does double duty. You can use it to lightly coat your pots and pans before cooking, or you can spray the oil directly on salads and vegetables. In either case, spraying instead of pouring saves you fat and calories.

Rice cooker: rice is a staple of a low-fat lifestyle, but even experienced cooks complain about not being able to cook it quite right. That's the beauty of a rice cooker, which monitors the steam heat to produce fluffy, evenly cooked, perfectly done rice. Most models have a keep-warm or warm-up feature. You can steam other foods in this appliance as well.

Salad spinner: with this handy item, you wash and place lettuce or other vegetables inside a strainer that fits into a plastic bowl. Then you either pull a cord or pump a button to set the strainer spinning. The result: fresh, crisp lettuce and veggies.

Steamer basket: this inexpensive metal gadget has hinged, petal-like sides that will adjust so that you can convert almost any pot or pan into a steamer. As with bamboo and other forms of steamers, this type will keep nutrients and flavours from escaping from vegetables.

Stove-top grill: a low-fat method of cooking that will give you the taste of barbecue even in the depths of winter. Its non-stick cooking surface requires little or no cooking oil, making cleaning easy. Many models can be used on either gas or electric hobs.

Wok: the deep, flared sides of this type of cookware give you a maximum amount of surface area to stir, toss and cook foods evenly, efficiently and very quickly. You can even stir fry with water or broth instead of oil, with little detectable change in taste.

Yogurt strainer: a mesh gadget that strains the fluid out of yogurt so that it's creamier and spreadable.

Stocking the pantry

Low-fat and low-calorie don't have to mean low taste. Seasoning is the key. One of the biggest threats to calorie-controlled eating is 'menu monotony'. If you have to eat chicken five nights a week, you'd better learn ways to make it taste new and delicious every time or you'll be foraging around for the Kitkats an hour after dinner. Use spices to keep the taste alive (see Chapter Ten on page 233 for lots more tips on using spices).

No one expects you to run out and buy *everything* on the following lists; you can just pick things up as you need them. Nevertheless, our ideal healthy kitchen would be stocked with the following:

Dry seasonings:

Allspice, basil, bay leaves, caraway, cayenne pepper, celery flakes or seeds, chilli powder, cinnamon, cloves, coriander, cream of tartar, cumin, curry, dill, garlic (powder or minced), ginger, marjoram, mustard powder, nutmeg, onion (powder or minced), oregano, paprika, parsley flakes, pepper (white, black and coarse-ground), red pepper flakes, rosemary, sage, tarragon, thyme and turmeric.

Wet seasonings, oils, condiments and cooking liquids:

Apple sauce (unsweetened), chicken broth (fat-free), chutney, cooking spray (non-stick), duck sauce, flavoured extracts (vanilla to start), hot pepper sauce, jams, marmalade, preserves, ketchup, lemon juice (bottled), lime juice (bottled), marinades (non-fat), mayonnaise (reduced fat), mustards (Dijon, green, English), oils in bottles (olive and one-nut oil eg peanut, walnut, or sesame), salad dressings (light, oil-free, and/or fat-free), salsa and picante sauce, soy sauce (light), teriyaki sauce, vinegars (flavoured, such as red and white wine, apple cider, balsamic), wine for cooking (one dry red, one dry white, one sherry) and Worcester sauce.

Staples – dry, canned, bottled:

Artichoke hearts (packed in water), baby cocktail corn (canned), beans (canned), bread (wholewheat or wholegrain), rices (such as brown, wild, basmati, arborio), couscous, barley, evaporated skimmed milk, fruit (canned in its own juice), green chilli peppers (chopped), hearts of palm (jar or can), honey, molasses, mushrooms (dried or canned), pastas (dry, in the styles you prefer), pitta bread (wholewheat), snacks (low-fat, such as low-fat crisps, baked tortilla chips), rice cakes, and non-fat rye and wholegrain crackers, sweet red peppers (roasted, whole and/or chopped), tomato paste, tomato sauce, tomatoes (whole, canned; regular or Italian-style), tomatoes (chopped up and flavoured, such as with garlic and herbs), tuna in brine, water chestnuts (canned) and wheatgerm (a great substitute for bread crumbs!).

For your cookbook shelf

No low-fat, low-calorie kitchen is complete without at least a handful of good cookbooks. If you love to browse the cooking section at your local bookstore, keep these tips in mind before plunking down your money:

★   If you're not an experienced cook, make sure the cookbook you buy has lots of pictures and/or illustrations.

- ★ Look for books in which each recipe has a nutrient analysis – that is, a breakdown of the calories, fat grams, carbohydrates, etc, per serving.
- ★ If the goal of getting everything done at the same time (entrées, side dishes, salads, etc) scares you, search for a book with menu plans, such as 'While the chicken simmers, wash and cut up the vegetables. . . .'
- ★ Check the copyright date of the book. You want a book that's new enough so that the nutritional information and the ingredients needed are up to date.

Coming up: Our recommendations for cookbooks with healthy recipes. If anybody asks you for wedding gift ideas, why not photocopy this section for them? Or suggest book vouchers as a wedding gift!

NB: If you have access to the Internet you may be able to get discounts on the following titles from some of the online booksellers; you will also be able to order books from the far larger range of American low-fat literature, including books on low-fat Latin American, Caribbean and kosher cookery.

All purpose

Good Housekeeping Low-Fat Cooking – Step-by-Step Essentials – Good Housekeeping Institute; Ebury Press, 1999, £19.99
The first in GH's 'Step-by-step Essentials' series – a collection of over 150 low-fat recipes appealing to all tastes.

In addition to the fat content, each one is accompanied by a nutritional analysis designed for the guidance of those on low-cholesterol or low-sodium diets.

Rosemary Conley's Low Fat Cookbook – Rosemary Conley; Century, 1999, £12.99

Offers ideas for all occasions: from snacks to full dinner parties; from vegetarian specialities to meat dishes of all kinds; soups, starters, sauces, puddings and cakes. Every recipe lists the fat and calorie content per portion so that you can design your own balanced menus. And there's plenty of no-nonsense advice on how to eat well, slim down and stay healthy.

Sue Kreitzman's Complete Low-fat Cookbook – Sue Kreitzman; Piatkus Books, 1996, £12.99

Containing over 250 recipes, the sections in this cookbook include soups, pasta, vegetables and vegetarian dishes, fish, meat, chicken, desserts and cakes. It includes recipes for low-fat versions of hamburgers, chips, roast potatoes, curries, pâtés, salad dressings, ice creams, fudge-iced chocolate cake and tiramisu. There are also alternatives to butter or margarine, and tips for roasting and frying the low-fat way.

Instructional

The Conran Cookbook – Terence Conran, Caroline Conran, Simon Hopkinson, James Murphy; Conran Octopus, 1999, £15.00

More than just a recipe book, more an encyclopaedia Learn about various cooking techniques and equipment from the measuring cup to the blow torch. More than 450 recipes, sumptuously photographed.

The Good Housekeeping New Step-by-Step Cookbook – Good Housekeeping Institute; Ebury Press, 1998, £19.99

More than 1,000 mostly mainstream recipes, 1,800 photos and step-by-step instructions that include estimates for both prep and cooking times.

Prevention's the Healthy Cook – Matthew Hoffman and David Joachim; Rodale Press, 1997, £12.99

The basics of healthy cooking without the frills. Numerous charts and illustrations demonstrate such things as the differences between cooking utensils. More than 1,000 healthy recipes.

General nutrition, dieting and fitness

Food – Susan Powter; Orion Paperbacks, 1996, £6.99

There is a lot more to food than recipes. This book explains: the truth about food and how people look and feel; how to buy and prepare low-fat food; how to eat and enjoy low-fat meals when dining out; and how to make sense of confusing food labels.

The Food Bible – Judith Wills; Quadrille Publishing Ltd, 1998, £25.00

This reference book offers valuable information on all the sorts of shopping worries that can face a food shopper. It covers the construction of a balanced diet; the 'superfoods' that protect against long-term illness; diet for different ages; ailments connected with diet; food allergies; healthy cooking methods; and safe slimming. The final section of the book contains 100 easy-to-cook recipes, created from healthy ingredients and cooked in a healthy way. There is cross-referencing of 100 recipes to suit numerous health and dietary considerations.

The Vitality Plan – Deborah Bull; Dorling Kindersley, 1999, £7.99

Lose weight, tone your body and boost your zest for life with this practical programme which demonstrates how the only way to lose weight permanently is to combine a low-fat, high-carbohydrate diet with the right type of exercise. Clear explanations of how to work with the body to lose weight allow the reader to formulate her own perfect fitness programme. Easy-to-follow guidelines and inspirational menu ideas outline the basic components of a healthy diet and there are plenty of suggestions for nutritious breakfasts, lunches, snacks and dinners.

Quick and easy

The Quick After Work Low-fat Cookbook – Sue Kreitzman; Piatkus Books, 1998, £12.99

Containing over 100 tasty low-fat recipes that can be cooked in a few minutes, this cookery book includes chapters on soups, starters and salads; meat; fish and vegetable main courses; accompaniments; and desserts and drinks. In addition to recipes such as duck fajitas, Chinese prawns and mushrooms with noodles, there are also low-fat versions of family favourites like fish cakes, salad dressings, pizzas, pasta dishes, roast potatoes and creamy soups.

***Judith Wills' Slimmers' Cookbook* – Judith Wills; Piatkus Books, 1998, £8.99**
30-minute recipes which cut out calories, fat and sugar while keeping in the flavour. International dishes include Thai Pork with Almonds and Creamed Monkfish Balti.

Special dietary needs

***Meatless Main Dishes* – *Great Taste* – *Low Fat* – Sandra Rose Gluck; Time Life, 1997, £9.99**
Tasty and quick vegetarian meals using plenty of grains and vegetables.

***Sue Kreitzman's Low Fat Vegetarian Cookbook* – Sue Kreitzman; Piatkus Books, 1998, £9.99**
100 low- or no-fat recipes specially for vegetarians.

Ethnic/regional cuisines

***Healthy Mediterranean Cooking* – Rena Salaman; Lorenz Books, 1996, £6.95**
Low in cholesterol and saturated fats and brimming with the healthiest of ingredients, these recipes come from the cuisines of France, Italy, Spain and Greece.

***High Flavour, Low-fat Italian Cooking* – Steve Raichlen; Viking, 1998, £14.99**

240 Italian recipes based on low-fat cookery techniques plus advice on ingredients and how to combine them in ways to maximise taste and minimise fat.

***Wagamama: the Way of the Noodle* – Russell Cronin, Michael Freeman; Boxtree, 1994, £10.00**

A Japanese noodle book containing 50 recipes for ramen, soba and udon noodles and their soup stocks and toppings. It also includes a chapter on health and topics such as the history of the noodle, Zen and Bruce Lee!

***Stir Crazy!* – Susan Jane Cheney, Nava Atlas; Contemporary Books, 1999, £7.95**

More than 100 quick and delicious low-fat recipes for your wok.

***Stir Fries and Sautés – Great Taste – Low Fat*; Time Life, 1997, £19.99**

A cookbook of recipes for stir-fries and sautés that are quick to prepare and low in fat and cholesterol. There are nutritional details for each recipe, including fat, calorie and sodium content.

***Secrets of Fat-Free Chinese Cooking : Over 130 Fat-free and Low-fat, Traditional Chinese Recipes* – Ying Chang Compestine; Avery Publishing Group, 1997, £14.95**

Fresh, healthy, tasty, traditional Chinese cuisine with lots of information on preparation and finding and choosing ingredients.

***Indian Cooking Without Fat* – Mridula Baljekar;
Metro Books, 1999, £9.99**

Leading Indian cookery writer and television presenter,
Mridula Baljekar, demonstrates how to create delicious
traditional Indian dishes which are high in taste but low
in fat.

***Low-Fat Mexican Handbook* – Earvolino Patric;
Sunset Books, 1994, £7.50**

This collection of Mexican recipes, ranging from appetisers to desserts, reduces the calories and fat from a
wide range of regional dishes. An appendix offers a comprehensive guide to the large variety of chillies to be
had, as well as a glossary of Mexican cookery terms and
ingredients.

Fish and poultry

***100 Low Fat Chicken and Turkey Recipes* – Corinne
T Netzer; Bantam Doubleday Dell, 1997, £5.99**

Special cooking techniques and quick and tasty low-fat
recipes.

***100 Low Fat Fish and Shellfish Recipes* – Corinne
T Netzer; Bantam Doubleday Dell, 1997, £5.99**

Reader-friendly book featuring preparation, cooking
techniques and terrific recipes.

Pasta

***100 Great Low-fat Pasta Sauces* – Maggie Ramsay,
Robin Matthews; Weidenfeld Illustrated, 1999,
£9.99**

A collection of healthy recipes for toppings to coat conchiglie, toss into tagliatelle or stir into spaghetti. Recipes include updated and light versions of classic pasta sauces as well as modern interpretations using low-fat ingredients.

Low Fat Pasta – Sunset Books, 1995, £7.50
A collection of more than 120 soups, salads, side dishes and main courses that help cooks to plan quick, nutritious pasta dishes featuring fresh and tasty ingredients. All the recipes provide less than 30 per cent of their calories from fat.

Salads/vegetables

***Jane Grigson's Vegetable Book* – Jane Grigson, Yvonne Skargon; Penguin, 1998, £6.99**
A guide to the selection and cooking of vegetables, from the humble potato to the exotic Chinese artichoke. Tempting recipes from all over the world to bring out the flavour and texture of each vegetable.

***100 Low Fat Small Meals and Salad Recipes* – Corinne T Netzer; Bantam Doubleday Dell, 1998, £5.99**
Recipes not just for salads but for soups and sandwiches as well.

***100 Low Fat Vegetable and Legume Recipes* – Corinne T Netzer; Bantam Doubleday Dell, 1998, £5.99**
Vegetarian main courses plus soups and salads.

Barbecue

Grilling – Great Taste – Low Fat – Sandra Rose Gluck; Time Life, 1998, £9.99

Recipes for meats, poultry and fish together with tips on different methods of grilling them, such as spit roasting and kebabs.

Baking and desserts

Sue Kreitzman's Low Fat Desserts – Sue Kreitzman; Piatkus Books, 1998, £12.99

A collection of low-fat recipes, including cheesecakes, tortes, trifles, ice creams and 'nursery' puddings; also sauces, fillings and toppings.

Secrets of Fat-Free Desserts – Sandra Woodruff; Avery Publishing Group, 1997, £12.99

Over 150 low-fat and fat-free recipes for simple-to-make cakes, biscuits, pies and puddings.

Low-fat Ways to Bake – Susan M. McIntosh; Sunset Books, 1998, £13.99

Biscuits, scones, muffins, cakes and desserts.

Entertaining

Blanc Vite – Raymond Blanc; Headline, 1998, £30.00

Here, multi-starred chef Blanc, in collaboration with physician Dr Jean Monro, combines use of the freshest ingredients with cooking techniques that complement the basic flavour of the food instead of masking it. In a passionate introduction, Blanc quotes Hippocrates: 'Let food be your medicine and medicine be your food', before going on to give his 10 commandments of food and be surprisingly (for a top chef) kind to vegetarians. Enticing, relatively easily prepared recipes for breakfast, snacks, fish, meat, veggies and desserts.

Champney's Cookbook – Adam Palmer; Weidenfeld Illustrated, 1999, £18.99

Palmer is the executive chef of the fashionable health chain and, like the resorts themselves, Palmer's recipes are distinctly upmarket – no bare lettuce leaves here. Instead, there's 'Chilled Roasted Vegetable Soup', 'Crab Cakes with Fruit and Ginger Chutney' and 'Fillet of Beef with Thai Green Risotto'. Palmer gives scientific explainations of why his food philosophy ('Moderation; Balance and Variety') works and suggests ways of integrating this into a healthy eating plan. The fat and fibre content of each recipe is coded with easy-to-interpret symbols.

The Art of Low-Calorie Cooking – Sally Schneider, Maria Robledo; Stewart, Tabori & Chang, 1994, £15.99

A book of 125 visually appealing, low-calorie recipes, including smoked salmon tartare, cassoulet, radicchio, orange and grilled onion salad, espresso crème brûlée, and prune and Armagnac ice cream. Calorie, fat and sodium counts are included with each recipe.

Recommended magazines

Give yourself a monthly boost of support plus a host of recipes and other ideas from magazines that promote a healthy and stress-free lifestyle. Our favourites are *Zest*, *Shape* and *Good Health*, available from all good newsagents in the UK.

Our favourite websites

The following have solid, accurate information about dieting, and/or nutrition and calorie counts, and/or fitness. All have links to additional sources of reliable information. The best of these tend to be US websites but the information they provide is largely transferrable to UK readers.

British Nutrition Foundation
www.nutrition.org.uk

American Dietetic Association
http://www.eatright.org.
Click on Nutrition Resources, then on Nutrition Fact Sheets.

CyberDiet
http://www.cyberdiet.com.
Provides a personalised diet profile and aids you in planning your daily food intake.

www.mynutrition.co.uk
UK website which offers free nutritional profiling and the opportunity to buy recommended vitamin and nutritional supplements online.

Mayo Clinic's 'Health Oasis'
http://www.mayohealth.org
Click on Nutrition Center.

Minnesota Attorney-General's Office 'Fast Food Facts'
http://www.olen.com/food
Covers menu items from many of the most popular American chains.

National Heart, Lung and Blood Institute
http://www.nhlbi.nih.gov
Click on Achieving Your Healthy Weight.

Shape Up America
http://www.shapeup.org
Especially click on Cyberkitchen.

US Food and Drug Administration's Center for Food Safety and Applied Nutrition
http://vm.cfsan.fda.gov
Click on Special Interest Areas: Women's Health, then on 'Losing Weight and Maintaining a Healthy Weight'.

University of Illinois' Nutrition Analysis Tool
http://www.ag.uiuc.edu/~food-lab/nat
Calculates calories and nutrients for almost anything you can think of.

Other good web stuff

Recipes On line

http://www.epicurious.com

http://www.kitchenlink.com

http://www.baychef.com

http://www.foodwine.com

http://www.mastercook.com

http://www.cyber-kitchen.com

Devoted specifically to low-fat recipes and living

http://www.cookinglight.com

http://www.fatfree.com

Miscellaneous

http://www.VRG.org
Website of the Vegetarian Resource Group.

http://www.caloriecontrol.org
Information about weight management and food trends.

CHAPTER NINE

Coping with Stress . . .

And Its Physical Souvenirs

Letters from nervous brides-to-be with knotty family problems are a staple of advice columns.

*O*ne agony aunt recently counselled a bride-elect whose stepmother insisted on being included in all of the wedding plans 'so as to show her "socially elite" friends what a wonderful wedding *she* threw, even though she and my father refuse to pay for anything'.

Not long after, a horrified advice columnist received a letter from a distraught young woman whose fiancé planned to place a large ceramic turtle at the front door of their wedding reception. What's more, the chap in question intended to attach a sign reading 'No notes less than £10' near a slot in the turtle's shell. 'I am appalled,' the woman wrote. 'He claims it is a common practice, used to contribute to the bride and groom's honeymoon, or for those who did not have time to buy a gift.'

These are extreme examples, but since a wedding is an emotionally charged event, and traditions, expectations and other factors vary among families, you should anticipate at least some family squabbling and stepped-on toes before the big day arrives (for help, see 'Ten Ways to Argue More Productively').

What it boils down to is the potential for more stress on top of the stress you may already be feeling as you run around taking care of the myriad tasks involved in putting on a wedding and reception. Too much stress

TEN WAYS TO ARGUE MORE PRODUCTIVELY

You and your mother/father/fiancé/future in-law don't see eye-to-eye about some aspect of your wedding/reception/honeymoon. Try the following tips from communication-skills consultant Audrey Nelson-Schneider, PhD, to keep the conflict from escalating and hasten a resolution.

★ **Allow time for anger and hostility to be expressed**. This gets the real issues right out into the open and enables you to manage the rest of the conflict more effectively.

★ **Begin on points of agreement**. Example: 'We both want to have the most beautiful wedding possible within our budget.'

★ **Remind the other person of such mutual interests throughout the conflict**.

★ **Don't deny the other person his/her feelings**. Don't say 'Mark, you have no right to be angry that I won't let you put that ceramic turtle on the front porch. It's an atrocious idea!'

★ **Actively listen to the other person**. Don't just be thinking up your next rebuttal.

★ **Focus on the other person's interests**. Read between his/her lines. Is your stepmother upset that you won't use her friend, the caterer, or is she really just resentful that you're not giving her a larger role in planning the wedding?

★ **State empathy whenever you feel it**. Example: 'Dad, I'd feel hurt, too, if my daughter walked down the aisle with her stepfather, like Mum wants. So I've come up with a compromise . . .'

★ **Demonstrate your willingness to see his/her side**. If you've *really* been trying to empathise throughout the conflict, it will be easier to see his/her side. Example: 'Mark, I can understand why you want people to put big bucks in that turtle – I know we need to get a deposit together for a flat. But among my friends and family, such a blatant plea for cash actually turns them off, because they consider it . . .'

★ **Agree with the other person when possible**. Even add to his/her argument. 'I can certainly understand why you want to go with Acme Photography, Mum. You know them well and you've had no time to research any other firms – not when you've been putting in 60-hour weeks at work! But I *have* had the time to do some research, and I am really impressed with . . .'

★ **Use 'I' statements instead of 'you' statements**. Don't say, 'Mum, this is my wedding. Stop feeling sorry for yourself and stop interfering!' Instead try: 'I can understand that things are a bit difficult between you and my stepmother, Mum. And of course you're more important to me. But she has done so much for me these past 10 years, and I feel she deserves to sit in the first row, too.'

can affect not just your mood, mental state and energy level, but your looks as well – by producing a new crop of pimples, for example, or robbing you of restful sleep (read: bags and dark circles). Later in this chapter, we'll help you deal with those stress souvenirs. For now, however, here are some ideas of ways to prevent stress:

★ **Talk to yourself:** if you can't avoid a stressful situation, try calmly to put your negative feelings into words, such as 'I'm upset because I'm stuck in traffic and I have a hundred things to do'. Then try to come up with at least three ways to make the situation more tolerable, such as 1) I can get off the motorway and take the dual carriageway instead; 2) I can buy a birthday cake for my friend Lucy instead of baking one; 3) I can call Mum and ask her to meet me at the bridal salon rather than picking her up.

★ **Use humour:** Stresscare, a Long Island, New York firm that conducts stress management seminars, recommends the 'blow-up' method of diffusing a stressful situation. You mentally blow a situation all out of proportion until it's ludicrous . . . and funny. If it looks like you will be late meeting the wedding co-ordinator at your church, you could tell yourself, 'My husband-to-be will have to meet her alone. Even though she is 40 years older than he is, they will fall madly in love at first sight. He will spurn me and marry her, and I will try to maintain at least a friendly relationship with him through the years by helping him clean her dentures, oil her wheelchair, and cook her mashed potato and rice pudding until she dies and I can have him back.'

★ **Think of delays as opportunities:** there are 15 people in front of you at the passport office and you have to be somewhere in 20 minutes. Always stash something constructive to do in your bag, be it proof-reading your wedding announcement for the newspaper, browsing library books for potential wedding readings, or writing thank you notes for early wedding presents.

★ **Make lists – but set priorities:** it's a good idea to make a list each day of things that need to be done. But such a list can be overwhelming if it gets too long. Solution: organise the list by making the first task the one that has the highest penalty should you be late in doing it; the second item has the next-worst penalty and so on. For example, the penalty if you don't 'Buy Mum's birthday present' is probably greater than the 50p you'll have to pay if you fail to 'Return the library book due today'.

★ **Set up a budget – then stick to it:** money is a major source of stress in life and weddings are a major expense. You can save yourself a lot of worry and head off arguments by sitting down with every-body who is contributing financially to the wedding and drawing up a budget: this much for flowers, this much for photography, etc.

★ **Delegate!** Gone are the days when the groom-to-be's role was simply to show up at the church on time. Lots of brides we know made their husbands-to-be completely responsible for planning the honeymoon or for making all music arrangements for the wedding and reception or for ensuring that all the ushers are properly attired. Ten to one, you'll be doing the lion's share of the work necessary for the wedding and reception, but to let him get off scot-free is setting a bad precedent! After all, do you want to be doing all the cooking and all the dish washing after you're married?

Family and friends will no doubt be pleased and flattered if you seek their help. But expect some resentment if the only chores you'll delegate are the unglamorous, tedious ones. If you assign your mother the tedious task of locating and reserving hotel rooms for out-of-towners, take her along and seek her input when you go to the florist.

★ **Lower your standards:** creating a wedding and reception will often feel like a full-time job. And that's on top of the full-time job you've already got. Something's got to go and in the weeks or months before your wedding, let that be something other than your wedding or your career. You will not be arrested if your flat isn't fastidiously neat or your nail polish is chipped.

★ **Learn to say no:** it seems to be a law of the universe that whenever you are frantically busy, the needs of your friends, family and colleagues increase propor-tionately. Your office mates are pushing you to organise the annual employee picnic. Your child's teacher wants you to bake 20 fairy cakes for the school fête. Your best friend asks you to babysit for her two toddlers while she and her husband go away for the weekend. You can effectively refuse without resorting to a scream of 'No! No way! Absolutely, positively not!' Just say in a harried, semi-hysterical, somewhat breathless voice, 'Look, I wish I could help but I can't. I'm simply over-whelmed.' Leave what you're overwhelmed by to the requester's imagination. You really don't owe anyone an explanation for saying no to a request for your time, especially if you know all too well that saying yes is going to make your life even crazier.

Stress management experts advise asking your-self a handful of questions before saying yes to a request for your time: Do I have to do this? Will I enjoy doing it? Is this project important to me? Do I have the energy and time to do it? If you answer no to any of these questions, seriously consider making that your final answer.

If you're Polly Pleaser and can't bring yourself to say an outright no, buy yourself time: 'I'll have to check my diary and get back to you.' Not only will this prevent you from saying yes because you were caught off-guard, it will also give you the opportu-nity to come up with an excuse for not accepting the person's request if you don't want to do it. You can then call the person back and say, 'I'm sorry, but I checked my diary and I'm busy that day.' And that's no lie! Because during this time of your life, you're busy every day.

★ **Give yourself a pep talk:** a lot of stress is self-inflicted, thanks to the negative and often self-deprecating comments we make when we're talking to ourselves, such as, 'There's no way I can finish everything I have to do.' Wrest yourself out of this state by overriding such thoughts with positive ones, such as 'I've accomplished a lot today!'

★ **Pet your pet:** University of Maryland researcher James Lynch conducted a study in which he found that just petting your dog or cat is a natural stress reliever. It slows your heart rate and lowers your blood pressure.

★ **Pop bubbles:** this is another somewhat off-the-wall suggestion but, believe us it works! A few years ago, researchers at Western New England College in Springfield, Massachusetts – yes, somebody actually did a study on this! – found that students were less tense and more calm and energised after popping sheets of bubble wrap. That's the plastic packing material with sealed-air capsules that you'll be getting reams of, once your wedding presents start to arrive in the post. Kathleen Dillon, PhD, the professor of psychology who directed the study, said that popping the plastic bubbles is in the same league as knitting, finger tapping and fiddling with worry beads – all activities that dispel muscle tension and pent-up nervous energy. She added that bubble popping has advantages over more conventional de-stressing techniques, such as meditation, because no instruction or practice is required to achieve satisfactory results. By the way, study participants preferred popping the larger bubbles over the smaller variety – 'a more satisfying pop', was the general consensus.

★ **Go for a walk:** a brisk, 15-minute walk has been found to be more calming than some tranquillisers. And regular walking – actually, regular exercise of any kind – helps the body adapt more readily to stress. A fit body pumps out lesser amounts of the 'fight or flight' hormones that produce stress symptoms such as sweating (see Chapter Five, of course).

★ **Don't bottle up your emotions:** according to the authors of the book *The Stress Solution*, repressing anger, anxiety, or depression decreases your resistance to stress. Get things off your chest. Having at least one close, trusted friend to confide in is also important. According to one study, women who are under severe stress and don't have somebody to confide in are twice as likely to be depressed as women who are equally stressed but who have a confidant.

★ **Schedule a music break:** researchers say that playing calm music in the operating room reduces a patient's anaesthesia needs, because it has a tranquillising effect. Whenever you have even a few minutes to spare, turn on your stereo and just sit, relax and listen. No rock, rap, or metal, please. You don't have to resort to 'elevator music', but do opt for something slow, non-vocal and quiet for best results. A woman we know, the mother of two hormonally berserk teens, swears by Pachelbel's 'Canon in D Major'. 'Canons', she says, 'are mesmerising.'

★ **Try a relaxation exercise:** here are three that we especially recommend:

● **Visual imagery.** Close your eyes and revisit the most relaxing place you've ever been to. Manufacture every vivid detail you recall – the feel of the sun on your back, the hissing of the ocean and so on. Try to stay in that place for at least 5 minutes.

● **Progressive muscle relaxation.** The principle: a muscle will relax automatically after it is tightened forcefully. Lie on your back and concentrate on tightening your forehead for five seconds, then relax it. Progress down your body, one part at a time, tightening and relaxing your jaw, neck, shoulders, all the way down to your toes. Try to set aside at least 15 minutes for this exercise.

● **The Relaxation Response.** Harvard researcher Herbert Benson devised this exercise because his studies showed that when people meditate, a feeling of tranquillity washes over them. In turn, muscle tension, heart rate, brainwave activity and blood pressure decrease. All you need is a quiet part of your home (even a closet, if necessary) and at least 10 but preferably 20 uninterrupted minutes. Close your eyes and repeat silently a meaningless word or phrase – you may wish to use the universal mantra *'om'* – over and over again. Try to concentrate on that sound only. If an intrusive thought drifts in, say 'Oh, well' and let it go. Then return to your mantra.

★ **Make your sleep as restful as possible:** as your wedding day comes closer, you may find that the amount of sleep you're getting is decreasing proportionately, what with late-night hen-night partying, relatives camping out in your living room, etc. You need an adequate amount of sleep not just to maintain a high energy level and a good mood, but also to ensure a fresh, rested look – one devoid of bleary eyes, bags and circles.

You may not be able to get the quantity of sleep you need, but you can improve the quality. Sleep researchers break the sleep cycle down into stages. The deepest, most restful sleep is found in stages 3 and 4. To get to those stages and remain in them long enough to receive their restorative qualities, make your sleep conditions as optimal as possible. Here are tips from sleep experts:

● Cut back on drinking. Alcohol does make it easier to fall asleep, but it also tends to make sleep lighter throughout the rest of the night.

● Exercise to ensure that your body will be as tired as your mind at night. Do your exercising, however, as early in the day as possible and certainly before dinner. Late-day exercising may make you feel too wired to fall asleep.

● Make yours a tranquil sleep environment. Your bedroom should be dark, quiet and at a comfortable temperature (most people sleep best when the room is between 60 and 65 degrees). Ask friends and family not to call you after a certain time – say, 10 pm, or turn off the ringer on your bedroom phone. Shut the windows and use a fan to keep out external noises (barking dogs, police sirens). External noises don't have to wake you up in order to disrupt your sleep. Such noises can kick you out of a deep stage of sleep and into a less restful one.

● Limit your caffeine intake. You don't have to cut out caffeine entirely, but if you're having trouble falling asleep or staying asleep, start by cutting back in the afternoon and evening hours. Make it a rule to not have coffee, tea, or cola after 4 pm. And be cautious even about decaf coffee. Four mugs of brewed decaf contain as much caffeine as a can of cola.

If you're using caffeine as an antidote to fatigue, be aware that while it will perk you up, it's only a short-term remedy. When it wears off after a couple of hours, you'll feel even more exhausted. Keep pouring it on and you risk caffeine overload, which can make you jittery and cranky. Bottom line: sleep is the cure for sleepiness, not caffeine. So, if you have the opportunity:

Take a nap or go to bed earlier: humans are biologically wired for one nap a day – usually in the mid-afternoon, according to University of Ottawa researcher Roger Broughton, MD. Studies show that napping will not only make you feel better, it will also make you better able to concentrate and to make complex decisions. The rules of napping: you need at least 20 minutes (30 is better) but no more than $1\frac{1}{2}$ hours. Shorter than 20 minutes and the nap will have no restorative benefits; go longer than 90 and it will be harder to fall asleep that night and/or your night-time sleep will be lighter and not as restful.

It's better to go to bed earlier than usual than to sleep later than normal: this is because we reset our body clocks by getting up at the same time every morning. Sleeping later than usual disrupts your body rhythms, leading to feelings of sluggishness or just a low-grade yuckiness during the day. On the other hand, going to bed early to make up for lost sleep has no side effects.

Vitamins for stress

You can't live in the real world and avoid every bug that comes around. But you can strengthen your immune system – your bug-fighting defences – so that you're less likely to be suffering from a cold or other such nuisance on your wedding day. Begin taking a multivitamin 3 months before the wedding. Take a basic, low-cost multivitamin – you don't need a 'stress formula' or one that's loaded with minerals or special herbs and botanicals. Foodwise, you should make sure you're getting enough of the following vitamins and minerals in your diet as these are the ones most responsible for a healthy immune system:

★ **Vitamin C** – The daily recommended dosage is 60 mgs, but 200 mgs is a better bet and you may need to buy a supplement to get to that level. Take any more than that, however, and it will simply pass out of your body in the urine. Good food sources: oranges, orange juice, grapefruit, grapefruit juice, strawberries, cantaloupe, red bell peppers, broccoli, kiwifruit and brussels sprouts.

★ **Vitamin B6** – Besides transforming food into energy and ensuring healthy function of nerve tissue, B6 is believed by scientists to help strengthen the immune system. You should get all 1.3 mgs you need per day through food, not supplements, because long-term use of supplements of, say, 200 mgs a day can cause permanent nerve damage. Foods that are rich in B6 include salmon, watermelon, potatoes, brown rice, avocados, turkey, chicken and bananas.

★ **Zinc** – Many women are lacking in this immune-system builder but supplements aren't recommended because excess zinc can inhibit the absorption of copper, another vital nutrient. Instead, strive to get the recommended daily allowance of 15 mgs through food sources such as split peas, lean beef, steamed oysters, shrimp, canned crab meat, wheat germ, roast turkey and black-eyed peas.

Herbs for stress

There are some herbal products that can help the body deal with stress. If you're taking other medications, or are planning to get pregnant soon after your wedding, check with your doctor first.

★ *Passion flower.* Taken as a herbal tea, passion flower eases nervous agitation, mild insomnia and nervous stomach. Your daily dose should be 4 to 8 mgs, divided among a cup of tea at each meal and one before bedtime.

★ *St John's Wort.* Taken as a capsule or tincture, it acts as a mild sedative for anxiety, depressive moods and inflammation of the skin. Your daily dose should be 2 to 4 grams or 0.3% total hypericin.

★ *Valerian.* Drink it in tea form to relieve restlessness, sleeping disorders, nervous conditions, mental strain and lack of concentration. Your daily dose should be 15 mgs, split among 3 or 4 cups of tea. Valerian is the most widely used sedative in Europe, outselling all prescription tranquillisers.

Stress-reducing beauty treatments

The week before your wedding, several superb stress-busters can be employed:

★ **Total body massage.** To unwind, schedule one 4 to 5 days before the big day – and why not schedule one for your groom as well?

★ **Hydrotherapy and aromatherapy.** These are relaxing options if massage is not your thing.

★ **Exfoliation, body scrub, mud pack, paraffin treatment, and waxing.** Some of these – ouch! – may only reduce the stress you feel about your looks! Schedule such treatments 3 to 4 days before the wedding so that any redness they cause will disappear.

★ **Facial.** In this case, too, you should build in at least 3 or 4 days before the wedding. That's so any flare-ups the facial may produce will subside.

★ **Pre-tanning.** Tanning is not a healthy thing to do, but if you insist . . . plan to get your colour in 3 short sessions the week before your wedding. Or try the new sunless treatments at salons.

★ **Manicure, pedicure, brow-shaping.** For best results, schedule these treatments for 2 days before the wedding.

How to foil mother nature

Stress leaves its marks. Here's how to minimise them.

When the eyes have it . . .

. . . puffiness and/or dark circles, that is. The skin around the eyes is the thinnest and most sensitive on the body. That's why the eyes reveal change so readily. **Puffiness** can occur when the muscles under the eye sag from fatigue or when the body retains too much water. Other causes: excessive salt intake, an increase in progesterone (the female hormone responsible for pre-menstrual bloat), or an allergic reaction to eye creams.

Many people wake up with puffy eyes after sleeping on their stomachs because that position allows fluid to gather in the loose skin around the eyes. The pull of gravity helps drain the fluid as the day progresses, but you can help avert morning eye puffiness by sleeping with your head propped on an extra pillow. Other ways to minimise puffiness: put your head back and place cold compresses, wet camomile tea bags, or cucumber slices over your closed eyes for 15 minutes.

We have **dark circles** because the skin below our eyes is more darkly pigmented than that of our cheeks, so our eyes appear to have shadows under them. Also, the thinness of the skin under the eyes allows the blood vessels to show through, adding to the shadowy effect. The degree of the skin's transparency is largely hereditary, but fatigue can contribute to the appearance of dark circles by causing the blood vessels to swell and come closer to the skin's surface.

Besides getting adequate sleep, the only real 'solution' for dark circles is camouflage. A friend – who insists that she's had very dark circles since birth – gave us her camouflage technique, and believe us, it works, because we've seen her with and without make-up. She applies a yellow concealer stick to the circles, covers that with her regular foundation and follows up with a second concealer product that is as close a match as possible to the colour of the skin on the rest of her face.

Cold sores (also known as the herpes simplex virus)

Obviously you need to avoid the external conditions that usually trigger your outbreaks, such as too much sun. But another major trigger in many women is stress, which we hope you'll be able to decrease and manage thanks to this chapter but that we know you won't be able to avoid entirely. Herpes is a virus, which means that antibiotics will not prevent a cold sore or hasten healing. Here are some suggestions for treating cold sores:

★ Witch hazel and rubbing alcohol. We've heard reports that breaking a cold sore and dotting on either one of these substances helps dry up the sore and speed healing.

★ Zinc. Some studies have demonstrated that a water-based topical zinc solution, applied as soon as you feel the tingling that a new sore is imminent, aids in speeding healing time. Zinc apparently keeps the virus from replicating.

★ Change your toothbrush. One study showed that 7 days after a toothbrush was exposed to the herpes virus, half of the virus remained, which means you can reinfect yourself. As soon as your present sore heals, throw your toothbrush away and buy a new one. Chuck out your toothpaste as well, because the tube can also transmit the virus. Rembrandt toothpaste offers a cold sore-fighting formula which may be worth a try.

★ Over-the-counter cold sore remedies such as Zovirax.

Acne

Stress throws your body out of balance and that can cause acne. The overproduction of hormones is what gives you spots. Some of us remember the days when acne sufferers were admonished to avoid chocolate and to scrub the face clean 6 or 7 times a day. These 'remedies' have been completely disproven by studies. In fact, washing too often can rupture plugged-up pores (the root of acne) and turn them into spots. There are ways, however, to head off a breakout:

★ Drink plenty of fluids. They help the body eliminate impurities from the skin. Water, diluted juices, milk and non-caffeinated beverages will all help you meet your daily requirement of 6 to 12 glasses.

★ Antibiotics. Spots are the result of the bacterial infection of clogged pores. That means antibiotics can kill the bacteria and prevent a spot from forming. Two weeks before your wedding, ask your family doctor to prescribe an antibiotic that is particularly effective against acne. Tetracycline is one antibiotic traditionally prescribed for this purpose and there is also a topical version available.

Taking an antibiotic will also help you ward off other bacterial infections (such as sore throat) that you may be exposed to in the last weeks before the wedding. A cold is a virus and an antibiotic won't help combat it at all. But the antibiotic can prevent a bout with a cold's secondary infections, such as earache.

The downside of using antibiotics is that they can disturb the usual mix of bacteria that live harmlessly in your vagina . . . and that can spell Y-E-A-S-T infection. To prevent that from happening, eat a daily cup of yogurt with live cultures – that is, not frozen yogurt! – or take an acidophilus supplement.

★ The birth control pill. If you're prone to acne and using or about to start using birth control pills, consider asking your doctor for a brand that actually helps to prevent spots.

★ Learn to correctly wash your face and use over-the-counter medications. 'Acne is *not* caused by surface oils,' says Leslie Mark, MD, a San Diego dermatologist. 'It's something that's happening inside the pores.' Mark recommends washing your face gently, no more than 2 or 3 times a day, with a soap that's not gritty and your fingers or a very soft clean cloth. Then spread an over-the-counter peeling/pore-unplugging agent over the entire area – not just on individual spots.

Probably the most effective and popular agent is benzoyl peroxide (one brand-Oxy 10). Besides its peeling/pore-unplugging action, it is also a per-oxide so it kills off some of the bacteria inside the pores. If you use benzoyl peroxide *regularly* – once or twice every day to the point just before visible flaking occurs – it can remove the plugs in 6 to 12 weeks and prevent others from forming.

★ Don't squeeze. Yes, you've been hearing this ad nau-seam since you first hit puberty, but did anybody ever explain the science behind it? Here it is: the more you squeeze clogged pores, the more they leak into the deeper layers of the skin and the bigger the inflammatory reaction (read: spot) will be. And the deeper the inflammation occurs, the more chance for scarring.

★ Get a shot. If your wedding is within days and you wake up with one or more of those huge, cystlike eruptions, see a dermatologist, who can give you hydrocortisone injections. 'The cysts will go down and your skin will look great,' Debra Jaliman, MD, a New York City dermatologist, told a bride-to-be in *Fitness* magazine. 'But it's not a long-term solution.'

Finally, an American supermodel recently told a *People* magazine reporter that when she gets a spot she puts a dab of toothpaste on it before she goes to bed. In the morning, she says, most of the inflammation and all of the redness are gone. Weird – but worth a try if you're desperate.

Irritable bowel syndrome

This condition is characterised by frequent loose stools and gas or by alternating bouts of constipation and diarrhoea. Irritable bowel syndrome is twice as common in women as in men and usually begins in early adulthood. It is almost always brought on or aggravated by stress. If you're prone to IBS and have a pre-wedding bout, try drinking 3 mugs of hot peppermint tea every day to calm down your gastrointestinal tract.

CHAPTER TEN

Dining on Your Honey-moon . . .

And Happily Ever After

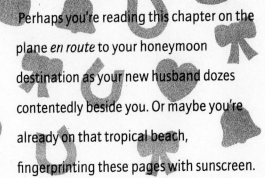

Congratulations!

Perhaps you're reading this chapter on the plane *en route* to your honeymoon destination as your new husband dozes contentedly beside you. Or maybe you're already on that tropical beach, fingerprinting these pages with sunscreen.

*O*f course you want to make the most of your extravagant and well-deserved trip away from family and wedding consultants. But don't let it go to your hips!

There's enjoying yourself, and then there's destroying yourself.

Use the following tips to ensure that the figure you arrive with is the one you leave with.

Honeymoon appetites

Breakfast

The lavish buffet/brunch offers everything you need for a weight-wise meal, such as cereal, fresh fruit and yogurt . . . along with every food known to stimulate the fat cells of your body, such as croissants, bacon, and big fat omelettes and pancakes. If you don't think you have the will-power to choose carefully, order *à la carte* from the menu – don't tempt fate.

A big breakfast eaten later in the morning should pre-empt the usual lunch calories. But what do you do when your tummy starts growling at 4 pm and your dinner reservations are for 8 pm? This is when you need that fresh banana you took off the buffet, or a call to room service for a vegetable crudité, or a trip to the hotel sundries shop for a bag of popcorn and a diet drink. Whatever you do, don't show up for dinner starving, or you'll just blow it there.

Lunch

Think about what you typically ate for lunch before the wedding and try to find similar choices.

When you're eating out three times a day, every meal can't be a 'special' meal.

Make trade-offs here that will allow you to indulge a little more at dinner.

If the only food available is the local fare of the honeymoon paradise you're visiting, it might help simply to stick to the basics. Make your midday eating a smorgasbord of fruits, vegetables, chewy grains and calcium-rich dairy foods.

Buy some fresh fruit at an open-air market, then wash and peel it for a sweet snack along with a small carton of the local yogurt. You could also order a chunky vegetable soup or garden salad at a pavement café, top it with some freshly grated cheese and eat it while munching on a few slender bread sticks. Or you and your new husband could pick up a small loaf of the local bread at the neighbourhood bakery and enjoy it with a chunk of cheese and a glass of wine.

Dinner

Extra calories can zap you from start to finish. There's the cocktail or wine, followed by appetisers, a first course, the entrée with fresh bread and butter and, of course, the dessert trolley. If you order something at every opportunity, you're looking at a minimum of 1,500 calories for the meal. Based on what type of restaurant you're in, or what the specialities of the house are, you should plan to order just what will be most memorable. Everything on the menu cannot be your first choice. Figure out what you absolutely must have and pass up the other options.

Workouts for two

Try to maintain your new fitness level by getting some exercise every day. That doesn't mean you're limited to using the hotel fitness centre. Look at all of the other fun ways to stay fit together: swimming, snorkelling, bicycling, tennis, golf, hiking, horse riding, even walking will burn calories. In fact, we know one honeymooning couple who were so entranced with the Colonial Revolutionary sites in Boston that they spent every day walking the 3-mile Freedom Trail. When they returned home, the bride weighed 2 lbs *less* than she had on her wedding day.

And don't forget how aerobically beneficial lots of sex can be! Look at the calorie-burning potential:

	Body weights	
Sex activity	110	123
Light effort, kissing, hugging	1.1	1.2
Moderate effort, petting, fondling	1.3	1.5
Vigorous effort, intercourse	1.5	1.7

Maintaining your new figure

All of us have read the letters in advice columns in which one spouse – usually the husband – makes a complaint along the lines of

'She is not the woman I married. In fact, she is twice the size of the woman I married!'

We know you want to maintain your new shape once the honeymoon is over and you return to the real world. Helping you do that is what the rest of this chapter is all about.

Let's start with a formula. First, decide the exact weight at which you wish to remain – probably what you weighed on your wedding day. Then go back to page 85 in Chapter Four and decide how much exercise you're going to continue to do each week. Multiply the appropriate 'activity factor' by your 'desired' weight. The result is the number of calories you can consume each day without gaining weight.

139	150	163	176	190	203
1.4	1.5	1.6	1.8	1.9	2.0
1.6	1.8	2.0	2.1	2.3	2.4
1.8	2.0	2.2	2.4	2.6	2.7

Recipe for real life: shop wisely, prepare creatively, portion judiciously

Maintaining your desired weight will be easier if you keep this basic truth in mind:

it is easier to control your kitchen than to control your cravings.

In other words, if you crave something that's not readily available in your home, you probably won't take the trouble to go to the store or the fast-food restaurant and get it – especially if it's snowing, late at night and/or you have a mud mask on your face.

How to produce the right environment? First, if you haven't already done so, set up a 'slim' kitchen (go back to Chapter Eight for the details). Next, convert your husband to the healthy lifestyle – or at least make him tolerant of yours and willing to make a few changes in his own. Some suggestions:

Hoisting your husband onto the bandwagon

❤ Insist on brown rice, wholewheat bread and whole-grain cereal as your pantry staples. If he whines, let him have a box of sweetened kids' cereal once a month.

❤ Make part-skimmed or low-fat cheeses your brand of choice, along with fat-free milk and yogurt. He'll get used to it, especially if he has no choice. If he's a big milk drinker, a good way to wean him off whole milk is by switching to the two per cent milk variety the first week, one per cent milk the second . . . and then non-fat for good!

❤ If your husband has a hankering for 'Mum's cooking', don't try to compete. Send him home to Mum to eat. Those nostalgia meals usually represent loads of fat and calories and you don't need the leftovers.

❤ Always serve a seasonal salad as a first course at home plus at least one or two additional vegetable dishes on the side. You'll both eat much less meat and pasta when there are more vegetables to fill up on.

❤ Bake or grill extra boneless chicken or pork cutlets and individually wrap and freeze them before the meal is served. They'll come in handy for weekend sandwiches, salad toppers, or as a fast dinner-for-one if either of you has to work late.

💗 While clearing the table, put the leftover vegetables in a plastic container and drizzle with light vinaigrette. Now you have a marinated vegetable salad ready for tomorrow's lunch.

💗 Buy quick-ripening fruit in different stages of readiness so that you always have fruit that is ready to eat.

💗 Stock up on enough fresh vegetables to use in the first three or four days after your shopping trip, then switch to frozen varieties or make another quick trip to the supermarket midweek. Overbuying perishable foods means you pay for it at the beginning of the week and throw it away at the end of the week.

💗 Make it clear what you want your husband to surprise you with on birthdays, anniversaries, Valentine's Day: eg 28-carat gold jewellery, theatre tickets, flowers, luxurious leather goods, perfume – *anything* but that dreaded 5 lb box of chocolates!

💗 Instead of keeping tubs of Ben & Jerry's in your freezer, agree to go out for ice cream when the urge strikes. Truth is, once you're settled in for the night, you're less likely to go out for those premium calories.

💗 If he must have his treats, buy individually wrapped snack cakes and pastries rather than boxes of biscuits or whole cakes. You're both less likely to mindlessly munch through a whole box when each serving is separate.

Your family + his family
= diet down the drain?

The size of your extended family obviously doubles once you're married. We're hoping that in the months preceding your wedding you managed to get the support of your own side of the family in your battle to lose weight and keep it off. Now, though, you may have to contend with a whole new crop of well-meaning naysayers. Some of your husband's relatives will probably have rock-solid beliefs about food and eating steeped in decades of tradition. Or they will not have kept up with the research findings that have come to light in the last quarter century that have been nothing short of revolutionary in the world of weight management, such as the importance of counting not just calories but also fat grams.

Your husband's Great-Aunt Beryl will probably continue to scold you with 'It's against the law in my house to eat apple pie without clotted cream' for the rest of her life. His Grandpa Ted will continue to bellow every time you walk through his front door – 'You're looking a bit puny, my girl! Well, we'll have to make sure we fatten you up today!'

When dealing with such set-in-their-ways people – indeed, even when dealing with relatively *enlightened* people – it's important not to come off as obsessive, preachy or strident. A friend recently confided to us that he no longer invites his brother John and John's wife Denise over for dinner. 'Denise whips out her calorie guide and fat gram counter with every course,' he explained. 'Makes the rest of us – snort, snort! – feel like pigs!'

Here are some subtler ways to spare yourself some lbs and a bad reputation while sparing others' feelings at family gatherings:

❤ When you're the hostess, establish your own signature style. Instead of being remembered for how much food you serve, impress your guests with how beautifully you serve it. Create sensational centrepieces, learn garnishing techniques, set a perfect table, illuminate your house by candlelight.

❤ Plan some non-eating activities for the family gatherings you host. Play charades or Twister, hold mini-concerts or sing-alongs, stage photo opportunities with all the guests, interview everyone on video for a recorded family history, set aside 15 minutes of every hour as adults-only time on the bouncy castle!

❤ Introduce some healthy and lower-calorie alternatives to the traditional family menus, featuring Grandma's heirloom trifle and Uncle Bernard's pork in cream sauce. Keep them all guessing what the secret ingredient is in your walnut vinaigrette dressing or curried vegetable dip and you'll always be asked to bring it again.

Consciousness-raising in the kitchen

Whether you're cooking for the two of you, for a gathering of family and friends, or just for yourself, here are more than a dozen other subtle ways to cut calories and fat:

❤ Take the skin off chicken. On a half-breast of roasted chicken, removing the skin eliminates 5 grams of fat, which is equal to 45 calories. Avoid self-basting turkeys when buying a whole bird, then baste with broth or natural juices to save puddles of fat and calories. Look for minced poultry that is labelled 'minced skinless turkey/chicken meat' or 'minced turkey/chicken breast' to ensure that you're buying a poultry product in which the fatty parts of the bird have not been ground in.

❤ Cut the fat off meat. When you trim the fat off a 3 oz (75 g) piece of broiled sirloin steak, you're also trimming off 9 grams of fat and 81 calories.

❤ Make it your house policy to use less minced beef in shepherd's pie, spaghetti bolognaise and lasagne to lower the fat and calories in those favourites. Stretch that 90 per cent lean beef with minced turkey breast or soy protein.

❤ You're much better off if your food is baked, broiled grilled, poached, roasted, steamed, or microwaved rather than braised, breaded, buttered, creamed, crisped, fricasseed, fried, or sautéed (unless you sauté with little or no oil). The difference per serving between the first group of cooking methods and the second is an average of 100 to 300 calories and 10 to 30 grams of fat.

♥ Beware of cooking oil that is freely poured into a skillet. You may find yourself using as much as 2 fl oz (50 ml) of oil to cover the bottom of a 12-inch (30-cm) pan with a half-inch of oil. That's 500 fat calories that can be soaked up by your food. Better ideas: non-stick cookware and/or an oil sprayer. See Chapter Eight for more information.

♥ Spice it up. Another thing we discussed in Chapter Eight is how seasonings can really liven up low-fat, low-calorie dishes. We included a list of suggestions for stocking your spice cabinet and you can break down that spice list into three general categories: the strong spices, with which you should use a conservative hand (such as a $^1/_2$ teaspoon for 3 servings); the medium spices (say, 1 teaspoon for 3 servings); and the delicate spices, which you can sprinkle on virtually to your heart's delight. The strong spices on our list include bay leaves, curry, ginger, cayenne pepper, mustard, black pepper, rosemary and sage. The mediums: basil, celery flakes and seeds, cumin, dill, garlic, marjoram, oregano, tarragon, thyme and turmeric. The delicate: parsley.

A couple of other spicy tips: dried/crumbled herbs are stronger than fresh and powdered herbs are stronger than dried/crumbled. Write this formula on an index card and post it inside your cupboard door: 2 teaspoons fresh herbs equals $^3/_4$ to 1 teaspoon crumbled or $^1/_4$ teaspoon powdered. Note that dried herbs need heat or an acidic medium, like vinegar, to release flavour. Salad dressing is a good place for them. Use fresh herbs in the salad itself.

And don't forget spice rubs – mixes of dry spices that you rub on meat and fish that is to be grilled, blackened, or broiled. Rubs provide intense flavour and they work well on roasted vegetables, as well. You can buy ready-made spice rubs or, once you become a little more spice friendly, make your own.

- ♥ Revise recipes that combine meat and vegetables – such as fajitas, stir-fries and stews – by increasing the amount of vegetables by one-third and decreasing the amount of meat by one-third. No one will notice the difference.

- ♥ For recipes that require milk, replace whole milk with fat-free milk. Non-fat milk contains 0 grams of fat and 80 calories per 8 oz (200 g), whereas a similar portion of whole milk contains 8 grams of fat and 150 calories. For creamed soups and sauces in which a thicker consistency is necessary, replace whole milk with evaporated fat-free milk. One half cup has 100 calories but no fat. It also has twice the protein and calcium of whole milk. Evaporated fat-free milk also comes in handy as a substitute for heavy cream in recipes.

- ♥ Reduced-fat sour cream instead of the regular version is ideal in sauces and dips since flavour and consistency are the same. Low-fat plain yogurt is another good substitute for regular sour cream in dips, but if you heat the dip, stir in a teaspoon of cornstarch per 4 fl oz (120 ml) of yogurt to keep it from separating. Ever try replacing sour cream with plain yogurt or strained yogurt (see page 82) when you're dressing a baked potato? It tastes different but delicious.

♥ Be prudent with salad dressings. A USDA study found that salad dressing is the number-one source of fat in the diets of American women between the ages of 19 and 50. Choose pourable salad dressings rather than the spoonable type in a jar. A vinaigrette will run to the bottom of the bowl so you don't eat it all, while the creamy versions stick to every leaf of lettuce. And do try the fat-free and low-fat dressings. There are dozens of varieties – you and your husband are sure to find ones you like. You can also use such dressings to marinate meat, to baste grilling chicken and fish, and to flavour steamed vegetables.

♥ Salsa! It's catching up to ketchup in popularity. Use it instead of the high-fat stuff like mayonnaise and sour cream. It's great on baked potatoes and as a 'cover' for fish or chicken instead of creamy sauces. And salsa is not only low in fat, the tomatoes and other veggies make it high in nutrients as well.

♥ Sauté vegetables in water, broth, wine, fruit juice, or cooking spray instead of butter or margarine which have a whopping 11 grams of fat per tablespoon.

- ❤ Take advantage of pre-packed salad greens. If you're sliding away from your commitment to eat more greens because you're too fatigued to wash and tear them up, bags that combine various lettuce varieties such as spinach, romaine and rocket are made for you. Just slice up some tomatoes or red bell peppers for colour, throw in some chopped green onions, top with a low-fat or non-fat salad dressing and you're there! (Great salad seasonings: dill and basil.)

- ❤ Substitute apple sauce or other pureed fruit, including the kind made for babies, for oil when you bake. Mashed banana is another substitute for oil when baking. Use twice the amount of fruit; if the recipe calls for a 2 fl oz (50 ml) of oil, for example, use 4 fl oz of the alternative.

- ❤ Use only the whites of eggs in recipes. Two egg whites equal one whole egg. You save five grams of fat per egg yolk.

- ❤ When serving cooked pasta, toss in a few tablespoons of the cooking water instead of oil to prevent sticking. If you must have oil, use a spray oil (once again, see Chapter Eight for more info).

- ❤ Watch out for 'fat-free' foods especially sugary things like doughnuts or cake. Don't ever believe that 'fat-free' means you can eat all you want of a food. Remember, calories are king! Some fat-free foods contain even more calories than the regular versions, because manufacturers have to add sugar and other calorie-laden elements to make the food palatable without the fat. A fat-free fig biscuit, for example, has 20 calories more than the regular version.

Some final pearls (or should we say diamonds?) of wisdom

- ❤ Never put off until Monday a diet decision you can make today.

- ❤ Weekends count! There are 52 of them a year! An extra few hundred calories in each one will put you in the next dress size by the end of the year.

- ❤ If you add just 100 more calories a day to your diet than you can use, you'll have eaten 36,500 extra calories by the end of the year and gained 10 lbs.

- ❤ Vacations are not an escape from reality, no matter what the ads say. Your real body goes with you and shouldn't come back 10 lbs heavier.

- ❤ Placing a mirror over the dining table, or above the kitchen sink, or on the front of the refrigerator – all places where you'll see yourself eating – will help you eat less.

We leave you with a chart on which to record your weight at every anniversary (may you still be able to fit into your wedding dress on the 25th!) . . .

. . . And our very best wishes for a happy new life together.

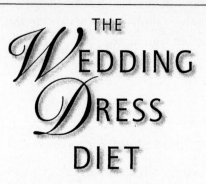

THE WEDDING DRESS DIET

LIFETIME WEIGHT RECORD

Wedding Date _____

Wedding Day Weight _____

Weigh yourself on your anniversary every year and record your married weights on this record. Use the space provided to make notes of any significant changes that may have occurred in your life that year, such as the birth of a child, loss of or change in job, moving to a new home, joining a gym or tennis club etc. Finally, take stock of your approach to diet and exercise and comment on what you'd like to do differently in the coming year.

Date	Weight	Major events	Self-assessment
_____	_____	_____	_____
_____	_____	_____	_____
_____	_____	_____	_____

Date	Weight	Major events	Self-assessment
____	____	_____	_____
____	____	_____	_____
____	____	_____	_____
____	____	_____	_____
____	____	_____	_____
____	____	_____	_____
____	____	_____	_____
____	____	_____	_____
____	____	_____	_____
____	____	_____	_____
____	____	_____	_____
____	____	_____	_____
____	____	_____	_____
____	____	_____	_____
____	____	_____	_____
____	____	_____	_____
____	____	_____	_____
____	____	_____	_____
____	____	_____	_____
____	____	_____	_____
____	____	_____	_____

Acknowledgements

In my 25-year career as a registered dietitian I have held many challenging and diversified positions in my chosen profession. When I reflect on all of the jobs I have had, I feel fortunate to have found work that I so thoroughly enjoy. Someone who understood just how much I loved what I did for a living once said to me, 'You got into the right occupation at the right time.' I think he was right.

Writing *The Wedding Dress Diet* was another exciting opportunity for me. But as with most new ventures, it could not have happened without the encouragement and support of others who believed I had what it takes to write this book.

The person I am most indebted to for seeing an author behind the veneer of this registered dietitian is Linda Konner, my literary agent. Of Linda I can truly say, she read me like a book. Her thoughtful probing of my experience and abilities led her to believe I had what it takes. Then all she had to do was convince me! I am forever grateful that she succeeded.

To Linda I must also credit the brilliant choice of co-author, Jackie Shannon. From opposite coasts we worked together like the keys on the keyboards of our respective word processors. I know I could not have met our near impossible deadlines without her cheerful coaching in the wee hours of my mornings and her nights.

As for my expertise on brides and weddings, I must first acknowledge my four sisters – now all married. I have had the privilege of playing a role on the day that each of them took centre stage and have amassed a wealth of dos and don'ts from those shared family ceremonies.

Next I must recognise the innumerable clients whom I have helped as they counted down the days until their final fittings. To each I owe a debt of gratitude for teaching me so much about what it means to be your personal best on this very special day.

And then for up-to-the-minute highlights, I must thank my eldest son and his bride-to-be who were staging the very last-minute details of their wedding day as this manuscript was being sent off to the printer. I could not have asked for a more up-front and personal experience in the long days and nights that I wrote these chapters.

May you all live happily ever after.

Robyn Flipse

I'd like to add my thanks...

To Linda Konner: not just your traditional agent, but matchmaker, firefighter, cheerleader and mother of great ideas as well!

To my co-author Robyn, whose energy, organisation, speed and creativity constantly astonished and delighted me.

To Jennifer Griffin, our editor at Doubleday-Broadway, whose never-flagging enthusiasm, thoughtful and concise editing, and rapid turnarounds of our drafts belied the fact that she was juggling other books . . . as well as attending to the million details of her own wedding!

To my daughter Madeline, for the interest she takes in each one of my projects, to the point that – barely eleven years old – anecdotes and titbits she collects through her own reading have ended up in every one of my non-fiction books, including this one.

To my 'hang-in-there' friends, Dirk Sutro, Reggie Calvin and Michael Vlassis.

And to Dr Eugene J Farmer, whose various contributions to my life since I became an adult go well beyond my own wedding. Thanks again, Dad.

Jacqueline Shannon